D0207215

MULTIPLE SCLEROSIS

By the same author

EVENING PRIMROSE OIL
THE Z FACTOR

MULTIPLE SCLEROSIS

A Self-Help Guide to Its Management

Judy Graham

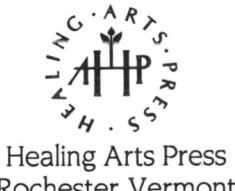

Healing Arts Press
Rochester, Vermont

Healing Arts Press
One Park Street
Rochester, Vermont 05767
www.InnerTraditions.com

Healing Arts Press is a division of Inner Traditions International

Copyright © 1989 by Judy Graham

All rights reserved. No part of this book may be reproduced or utilized
in any form or by any means, electronic or mechanical, including
photocopying, recording, or by any information storage and retrieval
system, without permission in writing from the publisher.

Note to the reader: This book is intended as an informational guide. The
remedies, approaches, and techniques described herein are meant to
supplement, and not to be a substitute for, professional medical care or
treatment. They should not be used to treat a serious ailment without
prior consultation with a qualified health care professional.

Library of Congress Cataloging-in-Publication Data
Graham, Judy.
Multiple Sclerosis.
Bibliography: p.
Includes index.
1. Multiple sclerosis—Treatment. 2. Multiple Sclerosis—Diet therapy.
Self-care, Health. I. Title
RC377.G65 1989 616.8'34 88-30103
ISBN 0-89281-242-7

Design by Irving Perkins Associates

Printed and bound in the United States

20 19 18 17

Contents

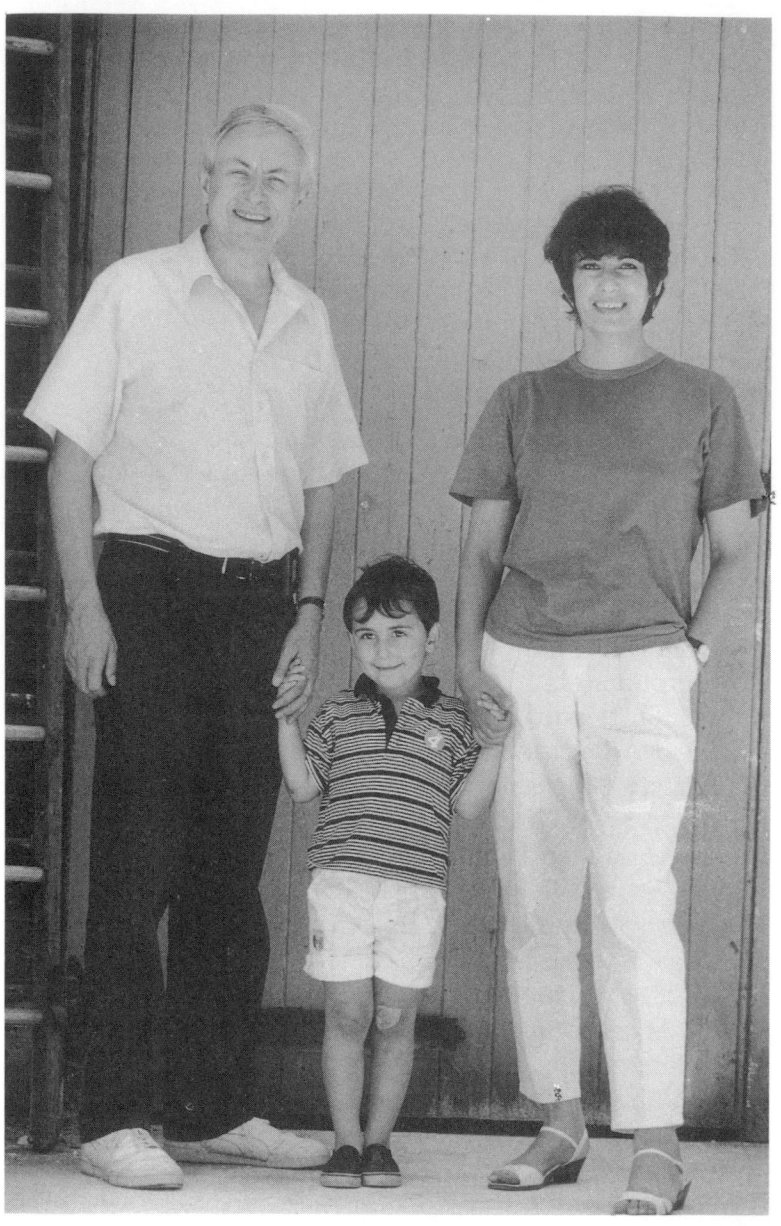

Author Judy Graham with her partner Dr. Michel Odent and their four-year-old son Pascal.

For my darling son Pascal

Le coeur a ses raisons que la raison ne connait point.
Blaise Pascal

Acknowledgments

This book could not have been written without the help of a great many people. Very little in it is original material—I have simply gathered into one place all of the various bits and pieces about the management of MS that have been written by other people elsewhere.

To credit all of those people would fill several pages. I would like to give special thanks, however, to Action for Research into Multiple Sclerosis, particularly everyone at the ARMS Research Unit at the Central Middlesex Hospital in London.

The inspiration for the book originally came from Joe Osborne of the Burton and South Derbyshire Independent Pool, to whom I give special thanks.

Many doctors have helped me with research material, books, and verbal advice. Some have written books of their own, which are listed at the end. Personal thanks are due to Professor Michael Crawford, Professor Roy Swank, Professor E. J. Field, Dr. David F. Horrobin, Dr. Jurgen Mertin, Dr. John Mansfield, and Dr. Patrick Kingsley. Two enlightened dentists also belong in this list—Jack Levenson and Vicky Lee.

Howard Kent, Lorraine de Souza, and Julia Segal did much of the original work in the chapters on yoga, physiotherapy, and mental attitude, respectively. Muriel Tristant did the typing while I looked after my little son Pascal or else looked after Pascal while I did the typing. This book would not have been finished without her willing help.

Last, my thanks to Pascal, who endured my putting him off while I worked, and to Michel, who has encouraged me in everything I do.

Foreword

This book by Judy Graham highlights the fact that anyone with multiple sclerosis can get better or, at the very least, can keep from getting any worse. Despite the knowledge that is available through the few doctors who have published their results, usually in a book for general reading, the vast majority of medical practitioners still see MS as an incurable condition, one that will lead eventually to life in a wheelchair for most sufferers and ultimately to death. That Judy Graham has done well with her own MS but is not medically qualified herself suggests that her advice is better than that of most doctors.

I, for one, believe in her approach, to which the majority of the five hundred or so MS patients that I am seeing at present, who are also getting better, will attest. Those who read Judy Graham's latest book will surely be able to find in it something that they can do to help themselves. The trick is to find out what is causing *your* MS.

When doctors do carefully controlled clinical trials, they try to apply the same treatments to one group while a control group has no treatment at all. After an appropriate length of time, the outcome between the two groups is compared and statistics are applied to see if the treated group did any better (or possibly worse) than the control group.

Although this is the orthodox way of carrying out a clinical trial and some would say that it is essential to *prove* that any benefit wasn't just pure chance, it often fails to demonstrate that the treated group did get any better. This is because there wasn't enough overall improvement for the statistics to prove the point.

If 25 percent definitely improved and the rest either got no better or continued to go downhill, the treatment would be considered a failure. No one would question whether those who improved had done so genuinely or not. The statisticians would say that their improvement was due to chance and that the treatment was of no benefit to the treated group as a whole.

The tragedy of this approach is that all MS sufferers are different. Their symptoms are different, their attacks and remissions are different, and some have the chronic progressive type and go downhill from the day of the first attack without any letup. So how can groups be compared?

Far better to find out what is causing your MS and apply it to yourself—never mind the next person. In my experience, an MS sufferer may have an allergy to milk, potatoes, wheat, citrus fruits, tea, or any number of other foods; a reaction to the amalgam filling in the teeth (but again some MS sufferers have had dentures since before their first attack); a gross deficiency of zinc or vitamin B_6 or B_{12} , which they don't use properly even when given large supplemented doses; or any one of a number of anomalies. On the other hand, only one or two of these factors may be important in your case.

I suggest that you read this book through quickly first, just to get a feel of what it offers, and then read it again, picking out the parts that you think could be relevant to you. Try to involve your own physician, who, it is hoped, will be pleased to do anything to try to help you, even if only to keep you quiet! Never give up.

My experience is that there always *is* a cause or causes for any ill-health, including MS. The problem is to find it. But you never will find it if you don't look. It's up to you to help yourself, and this book will help you.

Dr. Patrick Kingsley, M.D., Leicestershire
British Society for Nutritional Medicine
British Society for Allergy and Environmental Medicine

Preface to the New Edition

The origins of this book go back to 1974. That was the year when I was diagnosed as having MS, at the age of twenty-seven, although my first symptoms started a few years before that. It was also the year when the Multiple Sclerosis Action Group began. I, with a dozen or so other people, were its founding members, and we held our inaugural meeting in the London apartment where I lived at that time.

The group members all had one thing in common. We either had MS ourselves or were married to someone with it. Just as important, we were a group of very angry activists who were outraged and enraged that nothing could be done for us. So we decided to do something for ourselves.

Part of this book reflects the research work of Action for Research into Multiple Sclerosis (ARMS) over the last twelve years, particularly with diet, physiotherapy, and hyperbaric oxygen. It also includes ideas for therapy that have not been funded by any MS group, particularly those to do with food allergies, micronutrients, and prevention of MS in children.

Over the years, ARMS has funded scientists who have done some inspirational work with MS. The first was Professor E. J. Field, who at that time was in Newcastle. ARMS (at first called the Multiple Sclerosis Action Group) raised money to fund Professor Field so he could continue his valuable research into essential fatty acids, evening primrose oil in particular.

Shortly after, ARMS became associated with Professor Michael Crawford, a biochemist at the Nuffield Laboratories of Comparative Medicine in Regent's Park, London. His research, although quite separate from Professor Field's, seemed to dovetail nicely with it. His main research was about brain lipids and, with ARMS' backing, he extended his research to investigate a diet for people with MS that was rich in essential fatty acids and low in saturated fat. That research has now produced very positive results, which are described in the chapter on diet.

I was lucky—and forthright—enough to be a guinea pig for both doctors. My arm was proffered many a time for blood tests. I believe that my initials, plus some tables I do not fully understand, are published in some papers reporting their work.

Professor Field was testing what was happening to my blood as a result of taking Naudicelle capsules of evening primrose oil. Professor (at that time Dr.) Crawford was testing my blood for its fatty acid composition. The idea was to see whether a diet high in essential fatty acids would alter the initially abnormal blood chemistry. It did.

My visits to Dr. Crawford were always a delight. His laboratories overlook London Zoo and are right next door to the parrot house. It was not like an appointment with any other doctor. No one there wore white coats. I was on first-name terms with everyone, and at no time was I treated like a "patient." The diet that Dr. Crawford suggested shifted the balance away from animal—or saturated—fats to polyunsaturated fats. It was also highly nutritious. I was told to eat a lot of vegetables. This was the beginning of the ARMS diet, which Professor Crawford has since developed and finely tuned, and which has been used with such success by people with MS attending the ARMS unit at the Central Middlesex Hospital.

Over the best part of a year of sticking to that diet and also taking evening primrose oil capsules, my blood chemistry became normal in its composition of essential fatty acids. By Professor Field's diagnostic test (see page 9), it ceased to give an MS reading.

However, there is no doubt that I still have MS. No one, least of all me, is suggesting that anything in this book constitutes a cure. After thirteen years, however, one can say with some confidence that there are ways to control, or manage, the disease. I am one of a great many people who can testify to this. Some of these therapies, then, deserve to be called "treatment" for MS.

During the past thirteen years, I have not had any MS attacks. At the time of this writing, I work as a television producer part-time and as a freelance writer, and I am also the mother of a very active toddler.

When my MS was first diagnosed, I felt as though I were wearing leather boots up to my thighs while walking through a quagmire in the Arctic Circle. When I did have "attacks," I sometimes went numb along my left hand and arm and all the way up my face; at other times, both hands went very tingly and weak; at still other times, I couldn't feel my feet and could tell what kind of shoes I had on only by looking; sometimes my walking was horribly stiff and I had to hold on to walls and furniture to keep my balance across a room.

I remember sometimes coming from work and flaking out on the sofa, not knowing why I felt so lifeless. One nightmarish day I was faced by a flight of stairs with no hand rails, and I knew the only way I could possibly get down them would be on my bottom or on someone's arm.

Today, I do still have MS symptoms, but none that you would notice. I have given up attempting to wear high-heel shoes and find I can walk faster and keep my balance better with flat rubber-soled lace-up shoes. I can't attempt to run for a bus and have missed many!

I do still get cold feet and legs from time to time, have slightly weak eyes, and often feel that everything is an effort. Fatigue is still my most disabling symptom. Even so, I can still work and can push the baby's buggy for a short walk on Hampstead Heath—although I do find it hard to keep up with him when he scampers off at full toddle.

All that has happened during the last thirteen years is that my condition has stabilized, and I haven't had any attacks. I can't claim the spectacular improvements of people like Roger MacDougall or Alan Greer, who have been photographed balancing on one leg, waving from ladders, or cavorting along heathland or beaches.

Nor am I at the best end of the spectrum of people with MS. I know some people with MS who climb mountains, play squash, run companies, or edit magazines. I can do none of these things, although many people with MS would be quite happy to be as mildly disabled as I am fifteen years after diagnosis.

So what do I do to control my MS? The book describes in detail all of the things that one could possibly do to help control the disease. Some of them I have done, some of them I used to do or do spasmodically, some of them I have not needed to do, and some of them I still do today.

I have been taking evening primrose oil capsules religiously every day since 1974, plus a variety of vitamin and mineral supplements (for the full list see Chapter 8). Very recently, I have seen a doctor trained in clinical ecology, Dr. Patrick Kingsley, as he has had so much success with MS. He advised me to give up tea, coffee, sugar, milk products, and yeast immediately. Even though I had not felt too bad while eating all of these things, there was a dramatic effect almost overnight when I gave all of them up. It was as though a fog had lifted. I had much more energy and no longer felt vaguely ill all the time.

The more I learn about MS, the more I am convinced that food sensitivity and other environmental allergies do play a part.* This book reflects the research on low saturated fat/high polyunsaturated fat diets. If the clinical ecologists are right and milk is the number one allergen, it means giving up ALL MILK PRODUCTS, no matter how skimmed or low fat they are. Of all the foods I have given up, milk and dairy products are the hardest to avoid. But it is worth it.

I have fluctuated in my adherence to an exercise regimen, even though I am convinced that sticking to a regular exercise program is the right thing to do. During those times when I have done regular exercise or practiced yoga, I have noticed the benefits in terms of fitness, suppleness, and increased stamina. During my lazy periods, I have noticed how stiff and tired I am by comparison. There seems no doubt that gentle exercise, stopping before you get tired, really does help.

Recently, I had a course of hyperbaric oxygen. This did make me full of energy. As I had no real symptoms, however, it was difficult to see what benefit it had been to me.

For most of the past thirteen years, I have been treated by an

---

*For a definition of *allergy* in this context, please see page 95.

acupuncturist, who also uses osteopathy and homeopathy when needed. I have also had deep massage treatment from time to time. All have helped.

This book covers an all-embracing approach to MS. People sometimes ask me in exasperated tones how I know which thing is doing good when there are so many of them. The idea is not to conduct some kind of scientific experiment as if one were testing a drug. Quite possibly, the self-help therapies in this book work together as a total lifestyle.

Once you start researching multiple sclerosis, you very quickly discover that many people who are involved with MS, for whatever reason, back different horses when it comes to treatment or management of the disease. Some people get evangelical about hyperbaric oxygen treatment, others about allergies, others about diet. Once people become religious about their own chosen therapy, they think that they have seen The Way and The Light and that everyone else is wrong, misguided, mad, mistaken, and barking up the wrong tree.

It has been my privilege over the years to be allowed to flit from one evangelical group to another, thus becoming aware of why certain people feel very pro about the way of treating MS and equally anti about the other ways. Taking a broad overview, I have tried to see how more than one road might lead to Rome. I have been truly catholic, truly eclectic, in my approach.

As a journalist, I have been careful not to align myself too closely with any one therapy. Although I am a member of ARMS and the MS Society, I do not necessarily share their policy viewpoints, nor they mine.

All opinions and conclusions in this book are my own. I have no financial, business, or other interest in any of the companies listed in this book. I mention this because some of my critics have hinted that anyone who espouses the attitudes described in this book must be in it for the money. This is untrue.

If I were to nail my colors to the mast, I would stand behind those doctors who have done the revolutionary research on polyunsaturates and a low fat diet. What I find maddening is that this research began in the 1960s, yet even now it is still not used in the prevention and treatment of multiple sclerosis. I am also impressed by the work of the "clinical ecology" doctors who are having such success with food allergy techniques.

I certainly wish that a book like this had existed when I knew nothing of MS back in 1974. My hope is that this book will satisfy a sorely felt need, particularly that of newly diagnosed people all over the world. If doctors are failing to answer this need, then we must do it ourselves.

Introduction

Many people with MS are more disabled than they need to be. Many people with MS are getting worse, when right now they could be getting better.

It is truly a scandal that doctors wait for a patient with MS to become visibly disabled before making a diagnosis (if they make one at all). Doctors have some stock reactions to finding that a patient has MS. Some still don't tell the patient that he or she has MS, putting the patient off with some explanation for the symptoms. Others diagnose MS on the patient's chart but don't tell the patient. They justify this by saying that there is no point in telling the patient because nothing can be done anyway, and a diagnosis of MS could send the patient into a terrible depression or even lead to suicide. Another stock response is to tell the patient that he or she has MS but then say "Go away and forget about it" or else "I'm sorry, there is nothing we can do for you."

All of these responses are based on the doctor's belief that MS is a chronic disease for which there is no known cause, cure, or treatment. The result of this belief is that many thousands of people with MS are allowed to get worse. One could even dare suggest that certain procedures or treatments done in the name of medicine actually accelerate the deterioration of MS sufferers.

Surely the aim of medicine should be to treat an illness at the earliest opportunity, before it has taken hold, rather than wait for it to develop into a chronic illness? By and large, however, waiting is what is happening now, the world over, with multiple sclerosis.

The record of orthodox medicine in regard to MS has been poor. Other ways now need to be found. For too long, doctors have gone along with the received wisdom about MS—that there is no known cause, cure, or treatment. This received wisdom now must be seriously challenged on several scores. This book takes up that challenge.

My view in this book is that there are probably several causes of MS. There may be clues in the medical history, diet, lifestyle, stresses, and attitudes of each person with MS, if only we look for them. Many factors may be involved in causing MS.

If that is so, it is most unlikely that there can be a single cure for such a multi-factorial disease. I believe that the concept of "cure" is not helpful, as it is based on the idea that a drug can be a magic bullet, in the way that an antibiotic can cure an infection. I cannot see how this can apply to multiple sclerosis. Instead, one can think of recovering one's health and well-being, which I believe *is* possible. I believe that there are several treatments that can bring about this increase in health and well-being. I do not believe that any one drug treatment is ever likely to bring this about. The treatments, or management programs, described in this book involve every aspect and layer of life. These treatments may not have been rigorously tested by scientific method, but we now have enough studies and enough anecdotal evidence to suggest strongly that the progression of MS can be slowed down, halted, or even reversed.

The kinds of therapies listed in this book do not lend themselves to the rigorous double-blind controlled trials beloved of scientists. They are not drugs and cannot be tested as if they were.

Moreover, doctors are always saying that no two cases of MS are alike. If that is so, how can they possibly bunch together 200 or 300 MS cases for a trial, and how can they possibly match them against controls? This stumbling block has always baffled me when doctors start waving their "there is no scientific evidence" finger at me. And, quite apart from anything else, many people consider it unethical to deprive the control group of a therapy that they are convinced is of benefit.

It is true that nothing in this book can be described as scientific proof. That is what doctors are waiting for. While they wait, however, thousands of people with MS are getting worse and worse—many of them perhaps needlessly. If anecdotal evidence were not treated with such unjustifiable derision, and if the medical profession would take a more flexible approach and see each patient as an individual, see healing as an art rather than a science, and stop dividing the body into pigeonholes, thousands of patients would benefit.

It is nothing short of a scandal that doctors do so little to help MS patients. When you go to see your doctor as an MS patient, the doctor should be able to say to you, "Yes, there are many things that we can do to help you. There is a special diet that helps; there are vitamins, minerals, and other supplements I can prescribe that might help; I can refer you to the physiotherapist at the local hospital; you can go to the local gym; if you have any bladder problems I can refer you to a urologist who can treat them; I can have your blood tested for allergies; and we can run a yoga class on Fridays."

Of course, doctors may prescribe drugs. Corticosteroids such as prednisolone work as immunosuppressants. When there is a flare-up, corticosteroids work by dampening it down. Drugs such as this are effective in the short term, but I do not believe that they are the answer in the long term. Drugs like this do have side effects, which are cumulative. These side effects include moon face, superfluous hair, and candidiasis. Immuno-suppressive drugs also weaken the immune system.

The aim of everything in this book is to do the exact opposite—to strengthen the immune system without resorting to drugs. Effective drugs do not necessarily equate with good health. A recent study by the British Office of Health Economics raised doubts about whether the UK's high drug bill improved health. In a foreword to the report, Professor John Butterfield, Regius Professor of Physics at Cambridge University, said, "What matters in modern medicine is how much better the patients feel, how much more fully they can live their lives, and how much they can contribute to the wealth of society in a cultural rather than simply financial sense."

As things stand at the moment, the more usual picture is for patients to go to their doctor and mention that they are on a special diet or taking particular supplements. Although these supplements are prescribable, they are not easy to get, so doctors just let such patients get on with it, in a *laissez-faire* sort of way.

This book is a self-help guide. How much better our health system would be if patients with a chronic disease did not have to rely on *self*-help to *get* help. Doctors tend to think that MS is an incurable and chronic disease and that there is nothing they can do. I believe that when you put all the facts together—as I have done in this book—you have to reach the more hopeful conclusion that there *are* practices that can help.

After reading this book, you may decide to take a bolder approach with your physician and ask quite firmly to be referred to specialists who can help you. It is iniquitous, for example, that so few MS patients are referred to a physiotherapist *at a time when they can still be helped.*

When the MS Action Group was founded in 1974, its aim was to encourage medical research on MS. My own view is that the time has come to stir up doctors and convince them that they have an important part to play in the management of multiple sclerosis.

Self-help alone is not enough, but it does have certain virtues. It means that you decide to do something to help yourself, rather than have others do things for you. That decision to help yourself will make you feel much more positive.

Those who have been told they have MS should also be told that many, many people with MS have managed to stay well by following certain guidelines. Surely this is better than a sentence of slowly getting worse and worse, with nothing that can be done.

It cannot be guaranteed that doing the things in this book will stop you from getting worse, but the suggestions are worth a try. At the very least, this book suggests a healthy way of life.

For many—if not all—something *can* be done. This book tells you how.

1

What Exactly Is MS?

If you know what is going on in this disease, it is easier to understand why the self-help management program is relevant. The trouble is that what exactly *is* going on in MS is still not completely understood. One scientist recently described MS as "baroque in its complexity."

Thirteen years ago, when ARMS was first founded, scientists in the MS field of research were fairly confidently predicting that the answer to MS would be found during the next five to ten years. A whole decade later, however, the more that is discovered, the more questions are raised. Nowadays, one is not even quite sure how to classify MS. It has always been called a neurological disease, as the symptoms are mostly neurological. So neurologists have made MS their specialty.

But perhaps MS is neurological only in its manifestations. It now seems that MS is also a vascular disease, in which the walls of the tiny blood vessels of the microcirculation are weakened and breached. MS is also a disease of the immune system, an autoimmune disease in which various components of the body's defense system attack the very tissues they should be defending. MS also seems to be a metabolic disorder in which there is an inborn inability to handle fats properly. This would also make MS a genetic disorder. Hormones (particularly the so-called stress hormones) may also be involved somewhere, thus bringing in the field of endocrinology.

What seems nonsensical from a layperson's point of view is the pigeonholing of modern medicine into the different disciplines of neurology, immunology, cardiology, biochemistry, genetics, virology, endocrinology, and so on. Surely MS is an example of the interrelatedness of all bodily systems and of how unproductive it is to make a disease the province of any one specialty.

The jigsaw pieces making up MS become ever more complex. It would be possible to blind you with science and go on about immunoglobulins, abnormal IgG ratios, monoclonal antibodies, or histocompatibility antigens, but all of these pieces have not yet been put together, and they are not strictly part of a self-help guide anyway. These terms all come from the vocabulary of orthodox medicine. Practitioners of alternative medicine do not see things in the same way at all. Their viewpoint is far more holistic. They do not fragment the body into bits and systems but see the whole person—body and mind—as one entity. Any disease is seen literally as dis-ease. Alternative practitioners see each person as an individual and do not go along with the "scientific method" whereby any therapy must be submitted to a carefully controlled trial.

It seems to me a crying shame that anecdotal evidence is dismissed so disparagingly by orthodox doctors. If one took the time to listen attentively to all of the anecdotal evidence on MS (and there is a huge amount), a very hopeful picture of treating MS would emerge. Doctors are quite happy to use the empirical approach when it suits them. There is now a strong case for following the empirical approach with MS.

WHAT IS HAPPENING IN MS?

Some medical facts about MS have been pieced together and are for the most part undisputed.

Myelin and Demyelination

The central thing that happens in MS is that myelin breaks down. Everyone agrees about that. What scientists don't agree on is *why* the myelin breaks down and whether this breakdown of myelin is the primary event in MS or follows from something else.

MS is a disease that affects the central nervous system (CNS). The CNS is the brain and the spinal cord. In the white matter of the CNS each nerve fiber (called an axon) is surrounded by a layer of insulation, called myelin. Nerve signals cannot travel normally without this insulating sheath, and without myelin there may be faulty connections between adjacent nerve fibers.

Think of these myelin-covered nerve fibers as if they were an electrical cable containing many wires. In a cable, it is very important that the wires should not make contact with each other. To stop this from happening, each wire is covered by some insulating material—usually rubber or plastic. The insulation assures that the electricity in the wire goes to its destination without short-circuiting.

In multiple sclerosis, the fibers in the central nervous system develop patches of demyelination. The damage to the brain and spinal cord occurs in many widely scattered areas. That is why the disease is called "multiple"—there are many patches of damage. The damaged area becomes filled with hard material, or scars. "Sclerosis" means scars. "Multiple sclerosis" means "many scars." How your MS affects you may depend on the location in the brain and spinal cord of the scarring, or plaques.

It is the white matter of the brain and spinal cord that is damaged in MS, rather than the gray matter. The white matter actually looks white to the naked eye. It consists of fibers that carry messages from the sense organs—like the skin, eyes, and ears—to the brain. The white matter also sends messages from the brain to the muscles.

The white matter also links various parts of the brain. It is the "wiring" of the brain. This explains why your ability to feel, move, and coordinate is affected in MS.

Although many questions about demyelination in MS are yet unanswered, more is known now about myelin and its breakdown than was known even five years ago. Seventy to eighty percent of myelin is made up of lipids, which are complex fats. Myelin also contains proteins. (You will see later in the book that the best nutrition for MS is very rich in the kind of structural fats that make up myelin.)

MS involves demyelination *only* of the central nervous system.

The nerve fibers in the peripheral nervous system are not affected in MS. The myelin in both systems is similar in lipid composition, but the two types of myelin are quite different in protein composition. The other big difference is that, in the central nervous system, there are glial (special connective tissue) cells called oligodendrocytes, which are responsible for producing myelin sheath, whereas in the peripheral nervous system other types of cells do this, called the Schwann cells.

Myelin Breakdown under the Microscope
Scientists are now able to see clearly for themselves what is going on when myelin breaks down. They have identified in particular something called a *macrophage*. In normal circumstances, macrophages are goodies. They are mobile white cells in the blood that infiltrate into damaged tissue. They aid other troops in the immune system to remove debris and bacteria by scavenging them, or gulping them up.

It now seems that myelin breakdown occurs only in the presence of infiltrating macrophages. Under the microscope, these macrophages can be seen actually gobbling up the myelin. MS is called an autoimmune system disease because components of the immune system turn against the body instead of defending it. These rogue macrophages are part of the autoimmune process in multiple sclerosis. Why the macrophages begin to destroy myelin is still a puzzle. Other bits of the immune system, such as the lymphocytes, are thought to behave in a hostile way too.

Then there are the *astrocytes*. Astrocytes are the cells that form the scar after the myelin is destroyed. They are turning out to be baddies too. They produce enzymes which are a bit similar to macrophages in that they are garbage collectors—they clear away dead and waste products. These enzymes may play an important role in damaging myelin in an area of inflammation. This inflammation itself is a key part of an acute attack of MS. Moreover, the myelin contains an enzyme system of its own, which can digest myelin proteins and contribute to breakdown.

The switch, or trigger, that turns these processes on is still open to debate. In any case, some scientists hold the view that it is futile to look for any trigger, as the process of demyelination is a purely degenerative one. This means that the myelin itself degenerates without any trigger because it was never properly built in the first place. The building blocks for laying down strong myelin were faulty, and it did not have the strength to last a lifetime, as it normally should. The building blocks that lay down strong and healthy myelin are largely made of structural fats.

Myelin Can Regenerate
Whatever the reason or reasons for myelin breaking down, the heartening thing to know is that myelin can regenerate. Not long ago, it was thought that myelin could not regenerate, but now this idea seems to be mistaken. Although myelin is a relatively stable structure, individual components do turn over, with old components being broken down and replaced with newly formed components.

This means that some of the damage sustained by the nervous system is, in principle, capable of recovery. MS plaques may be not fixed sites of permanent damage, but areas in which damaged tissues are attempting self-repair. The trick is to know exactly what conditions aid that recovery. Some or a combination of the therapies featured in this book may be providing the conditions that aid myelin regeneration. For a long time, researchers have been saying that, if only they could find out what made myelin regenerate, they could solve the puzzle of MS.

Other Ideas about the Mechanisms Involved in MS

An Inborn Mishandling of Essential Fatty Acids
As long ago as the 1960s, a British scientist, R. H. S. Thompson, came up with the brilliant hypothesis that MS may develop against a background of inborn mishandling of certain essential fatty acids. This has been called "Thompson's anomaly." The significance of this anomaly is that the "soil" is prepared for the development of MS. Because of this mishandling of essential fatty acids, *all* cells in the body are abnormal, and myelin is built in such a weak way that it is prone to degeneration, falling to pieces rather like a badly built wall.

An Inability to Handle Saturated Fats

Professor Roy Swank, champion of the low fat diet, believes that bunching together of platelets—caused by a diet high in saturated fats—stretches the blood vessel walls. This leads to a loss of integrity of the vessel walls, and in time toxic materials are able to seep through the blood into the brain. Professor Michael Crawford, who is behind the ARMS low fat diet, thinks along similar lines.

So, according to Swank, MS is primarily due to an unstable blood emulsion from excess intake of fat in susceptible people. This susceptibility might be a defect in the red blood cell membrane or a plasma abnormality.

Breakdown of the Blood-Brain Barrier

There is now widespread agreement that MS plaques are associated with, and form around, very small veins—or venules—within the central nervous system. These "perivenular" plaques evidently form when the blood-brain barrier is breached.

Blood is not supposed to cross over into the brain. Potentially harmful substances carried in the blood must be kept away from the central nervous system. If blood does get across the barrier, it is toxic to nerve tissue.

The lining of the blood vessels that supply the nervous system—called the endothelium—has a special structure and way of functioning that makes it a barrier against harmful substances. At the same time, this membrane allows necessary nutrients and gases to pass through it.

A breach in the blood-brain barrier is followed by local swelling, the breakdown of myelin, an inflammatory macrophage response, and the formation of a central hardened zone of fibrous material.

Several researchers working in the field of MS have come to the conclusion that the primary event in MS is the breach of the blood-brain barrier. Therefore, this is the first event that should be stopped. The other events known to occur in MS, such as the breakdown of myelin or rogue macrophages on the rampage, seem to happen only *after* the blood-brain barrier has been broken.

Dr. Philip James, champion of hyperbaric oxygen treatment for MS, believes that fat embolism is responsible for the breach in the blood-brain barrier. This is explained more fully in Chapter 13.

Broadly speaking, several theories agree that *fat* is to blame for damaging vessel walls. There is also some evidence that other factors can weaken the blood-brain barrier intermittently and thus allow substances in the blood to leak through to the brain. These factors include

- stressful events
- fatigue
- fever
- emotional upsets
- heat
- injury

All events such as these provoke a physiological coping response, which includes the release of epinephrine. This brings about arousal and mobilization of bodily resources, part of which involves an increase in blood supply to the CNS. There is also increased blood-brain barrier permeability. Anyone who has had attacks of MS knows that stressors often precipitate attacks. Mercury, a nerve poison, can also get across the blood-brain barrier (see Chapter 11). The aim of some of the therapies featured in this book is to prevent the primary reason for the blood-brain barrier being breached.

SIGNS AND SYMPTOMS OF MS

Symptoms can include any or all of the following: tingling or a sensation of pins and needles anywhere in the body; difficulty in walking; dragging either foot; loss of coordination; loss of sensation or distorted sensation anywhere in the body; feeling as though one is made of cotton, rubber, or jelly; clumsiness; double or blurred vision or temporary blindness in an eye; slurred speech; an urgency to urinate or an inability to pass urine; loss of balance; unnatural fatigue; a feeling of tight bands around the trunk or lower limbs, which can be itchy; pain; vertigo; numbness; tremors in the hands and arms; spasticity of the muscles or muscles that feel like jelly; a feeling of extreme cold like frostbite in the extremities; feeling like a wet rag in humid weather.

THE COURSE OF MS

Usually, the only type of MS mentioned is the relapsing-remitting type, in which someone has an attack with full-blown symptoms, followed by a remission during which the person's condition returns to what it was or slightly worse than it was before the attack. Scientists have been trying to find out just what switches people into a remission. Many have felt that, if only they could solve the mystery of remissions, they could treat MS.

The relapsing-remitting type, however, is by no means the only course of MS. The other common type is described by scientists as "chronic progressive." In these cases, there are no clear-cut attacks, and the person just gets progressively worse.

There are some rare cases of a galloping form of MS, in which the person degenerates rapidly and dies within a few years. It is also possible for a person to have one attack of MS and then never have another and live to a ripe old age.

Doctors sometimes say that the first five years of MS are a predictor of the future. Those who have not become much worse in that time are said to have a "benign" course.

The aim of this book is to enable one to recognize and deal with the disease early, so that one is not faced with the horrible prospect of getting worse and worse, at whatever speed.

WHY DIAGNOSING MS IS SO IMPORTANT

MS is notoriously difficult to diagnose clinically, partly because MS symptoms can also be the symptoms of other diseases. However, there are new techniques for diagnosing MS easily, as soon as the first symptoms appear.

It is important to diagnose MS for the following reasons:

- to exclude the possibility of other illnesses that could be effectively treated
- to start a management program before the disease progresses
- to be referred to specialized therapists, e.g., physiotherapists, before the disease progresses
- to have an explanation for the symptoms you have been experiencing and to avoid the feeling that it is all psychological
- to have the information on which to be able to make future decisions about your life: type of job, type of house, number of children, etc.
- to qualify for benefits, such as disability benefits, if MS has already affected your ability to earn a living

WAYS OF DIAGNOSING MS

A Clinical Diagnosis

Most cases of MS are still diagnosed clinically. This means that the doctor makes the diagnosis after you have visited several times, each time presenting with a different symptom. Usually, doctors wait for several different MS symptoms over a period of time—often years—before reaching a diagnosis of MS. A clinical diagnosis does not involve tests. Some people think that this method wastes precious time waiting for patients to have further attacks before making a diagnosis.

Specific Tests for MS

Over the last few years, certain diagnostic tests have been developed for MS. The least invasive is called the red cell mobility test, or the electrophoretic mobility test. This was devised originally by Professor E. J. Field. Put simply, the red blood cells of people with suspected MS are subjected to a test that measures how fast they travel in a certain solution. Red blood cells are abnormal in people with MS.

The red blood cells of people with MS are abnormal in their fatty acid composition. In Field's test, these red blood cells move more slowly than those from normal people or people with other neurological diseases. The test is specific for MS. Professor Field believes that this test should be done as soon as possible—after the first symptom of MS—so that treatment with evening primrose oil can be started without delay. The red cell mobility test is also diagnostic for susceptible individuals who have not yet shown any symptoms of MS (see Chapter 17).

Another new diagnostic test looks at immunoglobulin estimations in MS. It has been found that there is an abnormal IgG ratio in 54.5 percent of people who have MS.

New electrophysiology tests can measure how long it takes for a message evoked by stimulating a section of the central nervous system by use of a magnetic field to reach the target muscle. Researchers have already found that it takes longer for a message to get through in people with MS. In scientific language, this is called an "electrophysiological deficit in MS."

Scans

The great new hope for diagnosing MS is the use of scans. The main types are CT scans—computed axial tomography; MRI scans—magnetic resonance imaging; and PET scans—positron emission tomography.

Scanners produce high resolution cross-sections of selected parts of the body. They are safe and comparatively noninvasive and can provide detailed information about the brain.

Scanners have the advantage of being able to detect plaques and abnormalities in the brain and spinal cord. Normally, it would not be possible to invade these areas in a living person. With the aid of a scan, a doctor is able to pinpoint very specific tissue damage, such as plaques, swelling, and atrophy.

As well as being able to pinpoint damage from a diagnostic point of view, scanners have a huge potential in being able to monitor the effectiveness of any treatment. Before and after scans on people undergoing a particular therapy should yield useful information.

However, the trouble with all of these scanners is that they are expensive and not available everywhere. At the moment scans are a long way from being the standard method of MS diagnosis, of confirming diagnosis, or of monitoring treatments.

Standard Neurological Tests

A lumbar puncture can detect whether there is any myelin debris in the spinal fluid. This test is highly invasive and unpleasant. Many people report both short- and long-term aftereffects. With the patient under local anesthetic, a needle is inserted into the lumbar area of the spinal cord, and some fluid is removed for analysis. Some people are left with a truly dreadful headache— so bad that they can't lift their heads off the pillow—for days afterwards.

Neurological units can also give the visual evoked response test, which tests the eyes. There are also tests for balance, sensation, reflexes, and other neurological signs.

THE IMPORTANCE OF EARLY DIAGNOSIS

If you are not happy with just a clinical diagnosis or have not been given any diagnosis at all, ask to be referred for any or all of the just-described diagnostic tests. It is important to know for certain whether you have MS.

I think that very early diagnosis is essential, from both a practical and an ethical point of view, because I believe that there are effective ways of controlling MS, and the sooner you start, the less likely you are to get worse. In addition, there is now some scientific evidence that taking supplements of polyunsaturated oils can stabilize MS in the recently diagnosed (see page 41).

WHO GETS MS?

The usual statistic about MS is that 50,000 people suffer from it in the UK. This is probably a gross underestimation.

I do not know how these figures are gleaned. What is certain, however, is that the words "multiple sclerosis" are less likely to appear on a death certificate than an immediate cause of death, such as septicemia, for example. In many cases, patients with multiple sclerosis are not given a diagnosis of MS, so "multiple sclerosis" may not be on the medical chart. Both of these factors would lead to an underestimate of the true numbers with MS.

The mean age for a first attack of MS is about 30. However, it can happen as early as the teens (or perhaps even earlier) or as late as the fifties, or anywhere in between. Nonetheless, MS is called a disease of young adults. It is more common in women than in men.

MS is twenty times more common in northern Europe and America than in Africa. Studies show that the risk of MS is determined by exposure to an environmental factor during adolescence. People who emigrate before the age of 15 run the same risk of getting MS as the local inhabitants of the place to which they move.

2

The Management of Multiple Sclerosis

Here you are, landed with a disease with no known cause, no known cure, and no recognized treatment. You could languish in a private hell and lament your terrible lot, or you could decide to do everything in your power to fight the disease and help yourself.

THE SELF-HELP MANAGEMENT ARMORY

The full armory of weapons with which to wage war on MS includes all of the following:

- eating a healthy, low fat diet, rich in essential fatty acids (see Chapter 6)
- supplementing your diet with essential fatty acids
- supplementing your diet with vitamins, minerals, and trace elements, and amino acids
- testing yourself for food and other allergies and excluding substances toxic to you
- doing regular exercise, physiotherapy, or yoga
- maintaining a positive attitude to life
- keeping your brain active and stimulated
- getting enough rest
- avoiding fatigue
- leading a stress-free life, or as nearly stress-free as possible
- having satisfying relationships with other people
- resisting aggressive drugs that weaken the immune system

Even if you can manage only the first three all of the time and the others some of the time, you would be doing a lot toward keeping yourself as fit and healthy as possible.

Make an Early Start

Start the management program as soon as you are diagnosed. Resist being given corticosteroid drugs. The earlier you start, the better. Studies have shown that people who benefit most from this self-help regimen are the recently diagnosed. Don't wait until you get worse before you decide to try this self-help program. Use it as an insurance policy to help prevent you from getting worse.

It is *not* a cure. It is not a recognized treatment. The best one can hope for at the moment is *management* of the disease. This program can't do you any harm and it might do you some good. It gives you a chance of enjoying life fully—even though you have MS.

The Rationale behind this Management Program

Having read the previous chapter, you have an idea of what is going wrong in MS. Knowing this helps explain the various objectives of the self-help management program.

Why a Low Fat Diet?

- Because too much saturated fat in the diet may weaken the blood vessel walls and cause a breach of the blood-brain barrier
- Because shifting your fat intake to polyunsaturated fats will help strengthen blood vessel walls
- Because myelin is largely made up of lipids, i.e., polyunsaturated fats, as is the brain
- Because in MS the central nervous system is under attack; polyunsaturated fats are needed for the growth and repair of nervous tissue and for the maintenance of its structure

- Because MS is most prevalent in those parts of the world where a lot of dairy produce is eaten and least prevalent in those parts of the world where people eat more fish and more vegetable oils

Why Supplement Your Diet with Essential Fatty Acids?

- For all of the above reasons
- Because people with MS have been found to be low in some essential fatty acids
- Just in case your diet does not provide enough

Why Supplement Your Diet with Vitamins and Minerals?

- Because they help boost the immune system
- Because you need certain vitamins and minerals to act as collaborators if you are eating a diet rich in essential fatty acids
- Because your present diet may be low in vitamins and minerals
- Because people with MS may be low in certain vitamins and minerals, especially B_6 and zinc
- Because you need to have an optimal nutritional status to be as healthy as possible
- Because the amalgam fillings in your teeth may be seeping tiny amounts of mercury, and certain vitamins and minerals will help detoxify the body

Why Test Yourself for Food Allergies?

- Because many people with MS have allergies to certain foods
- Because these foods are toxic to those individuals and can make MS symptoms worse
- Because everyone is different and you have to test yourself to see which particular foods and chemicals you are allergic to
- Because many people with MS who have excluded the foods they are allergic to have improved as a result of doing so

Why Do Regular Exercise, or Physical Therapy, or Yoga?

- To maintain fitness
- To maintain suppleness and build up stamina
- To keep maximal use of your body
- To be able to do all your usual daily activities
- To have more energy
- To keep your body from getting stuck in the wrong postures
- To feel better and look better
- To reduce anxiety and stress
- To help calm the mind

Why Resist Corticosteroids and Other Aggressive Drugs?

The standard treatment for attacks of MS is corticosteroid drugs. They work effectively in alleviating the symptoms of MS and succeed well in getting people back on their feet because they are powerful anti-inflammatory agents.

So, if they work so well, why should you not take them? These drugs *weaken* the immune system. With each course of corticosteroid drugs, the immune system is weakened still further.

The self-help management program of a diet high in polyunsaturates plus selected vitamins, minerals, and trace elements plus excluding allergic foods does the exact opposite. Its aim is to *boost* the immune system. The more you strengthen the immune system, the more your body can heal itself.

Herein lies the crux of the difference between the orthodox approach and the approach taken by this book. You must choose between weakening your immune system with drugs that work well in the short term and a nutritional therapy that will boost your immune system but without immediate results or instant symptomatic relief.

In the long term, corticosteroid drugs also have side effects, such as weight gain, "moon" face, and unwanted hair. Immunosuppressive drugs such as cyclosporin have a wide range of bad side effects, including hypertension, swelling of the lymph nodes, and sometimes cancer.

All of the other things in the self-help management program are self-explanatory. Leading a stress-free life and avoiding fatigue are particularly important when you know how much stress and fatigue can precipitate attacks.

It's a good idea to try to incorporate all of these things into your normal life, rather than to let them take over your life like some manic hobby. MS is a fact of life, but it is not your whole life. Don't let it take you over. Overcome it before it overcomes you.

3

The Links between What You Eat and MS

Nutrition has had the best results so far of any kind of therapy in controlling multiple sclerosis. The more research that is done, the more certain the benefits of nutrition become. Nutrition is an umbrella word that can include the food you eat, nutrients in the form of supplements, and foods to which you may be allergic or sensitive.

These are the essential points about nutritional therapy for MS:

1. Cut down drastically on saturated fat, found in animal fats, dairy produce, and hard fats.
2. Increase your intake considerably of polyunsaturated fats—not just in spreads and oils, but also in foods like fish, liver, and green leafy vegetables. This will give you a diet high in essential fatty acids.

   Saturated fats and polyunsaturated fats work against each other in many respects, so you need to cut back on how much saturated fat you eat if you are going to increase your intake of polyunsaturated fatty acids (PUFAs for short). That way, you will get maximal benefit (see chapter 6).
3. Find out to which foods and substances you personally are sensitive or allergic. These may be surprisingly benign foods (e.g., apples or tomatoes), although the most common food to which MS people are allergic is milk. Cut out completely all foods and substances to which you are found to be allergic.
4. Eat a diet that gives you the best nutrition possible. Cut out junk foods and convenience foods. Always try to eat fresh

foods rather than foods that have been processed and packaged. Cut out or down on foods that only give empty calories, such as sugar.

5. Take supplements of evening primrose oil and fish oils. This guarantees you a good intake of the essential fatty acids needed for many vital processes in your body to work properly.
6. Take supplements of certain vitamins, minerals, and trace elements. Your body may be short of these, and they are needed to go hand in hand with the essential fatty acids.

The next six chapters go into each of these points in detail.

CLUES TO THE LINKS BETWEEN NUTRITION AND MS

Researchers in multiple sclerosis have to be a bit like detectives. They have to search for clues, piece them together, and find the culprits.

The Geographical Distribution of MS

One of the most marked features of MS is its geographical distribution. MS is a disease of temperate zones and is virtually nonexistent in the tropics. There are obviously a great many differences between life in temperate countries and that in tropical countries, but the key difference seems to be the food that people eat.

In those places where MS is most prevalent, people eat a lot of dairy produce. In those places where MS occurrence is lowest, people eat more fish and vegetable oils. The difference between an area of high MS and low MS can be as little as a few miles. Some of the starkest contrasts in MS occurrence are within Norway, comparing inland farming areas (where dairy farming is practiced and where MS is high) with coastal areas (where people eat more fish and MS is low). There is a similar story in some Scottish islands, where the rates of MS can fluctuate from very high to very low according to the main diet of the local people— high in areas of dairy farming and low in fishing areas.

Interestingly, a world map of the distribution of MS can also be interpreted in a slightly different way. The areas of high MS would also be the areas of high dental caries, which suggests that people had been eating a lot of sugar and have probably had fillings put in their teeth (see Chapter 10).

One of the first doctors to look at the world map of MS was Professor Roy Swank, now based in Portland, Oregon. He first developed his famous Swank low fat diet in 1948.

As a clever detective, Swank noticed several important clues. First, the amount of saturated fat in a typical American diet was rising dramatically. This was because there were improvements in the processing of dairy foods, beef cattle were made fatter so farmers could make more money, and processing techniques meant that vegetable oils changed from their natural states into margarines rich in saturated fat.

As the consumption of saturated fat has increased, so the incidence of certain diseases has increased—particularly multiple sclerosis, heart disease, and strokes. A link between a high fat diet and these diseases seemed probable.

During World War II, there were more clues for any medical detectives on the lookout. It was noticed that young American soldiers who had died of heart attacks during training and battle showed a greater degree of hardening of the arteries than their Asian counterparts, who ate mostly vegetables and rice.

In occupied Norway, fat consumption fell by 50 percent during food shortages. At the same time, there were significant reductions in death rates from heart attacks, and the rate of multiple sclerosis dropped too. After the war, however, fat intake and heart disease returned to their previous rates.

As long ago as 1950, Swank wrote:

> . . . possibly the incidence of the disease (MS) in entire populations may be related directly to the dietary fat—a high fat diet is not the cause of multiple sclerosis even though it may contribute to a high incidence of the disease by accelerating it in susceptible individuals.

Swank began his historic studies on low fat diet for MS on the following hypothesis:

The three-fold increase in fat intake in the past 200 years in the western world has caused a breakdown in the ability of the blood to maintain the fat and other matter in an emulsified state. The emulsion breaks down; the formed elements in the blood aggregate; and micro-embolism of the micro-circulation with consequent breakdown in the blood-brain barrier follow.[1]

In the UK, 40 percent of our diet is saturated fat. Around the world, tipping the balance of saturated/unsaturated fat in favor of saturated fats has coincided with increases in MS and also in cardiovascular (heart and stroke) diseases.

How Our Diet Has Changed over the Last Two Centuries

Nutritionists like Professor Michael Crawford have made a special study of how the food we eat has altered over the centuries. There have been profound changes in our diet in the last two centuries. During that time, the whole nature of the biological food chain has changed radically.

The biggest changes have been in fat and sugar. Humans used to eat meat from wild game, which was very lean meat rich in structural fats. Since the introduction of modern farming, however, animals have been reared to have stores of fat, which are full of saturated fat. The amount of sugar we eat has increased enormously during the same period.

Some people believe that humans were not designed to thrive on a high saturated fat plus high sugar diet. The rise in chronic disease coincides with these radical changes in diet in the western world.

The old-fashioned way of looking at a person's nutritional needs was to divide all foods simply into the basic food groups of proteins, carbohydrates, and fats. The emphasis has been on calories and energy rather than on cellular development. It is now obvious that the typical western diet includes the *wrong kind of fats*. What we need to do now is to stop going down the wrong road, do a U-turn, and take another route.

The Composition of the Brain, the Nervous System, and Cell Membranes

The next big clue about nutrition and MS comes from a knowledge of what the brain, the nervous system, and cell membranes are made of. One of the detectives in this field has been Professor Michael Crawford, who has made a special study of brain growth. He devised the successful ARMS diet in 1978.

His rationale for the low fat diet was based partly on the MS map of the world and partly on how the brain is put together. Roughly 60 percent of the brain is made of structural fats. These special fats, called phosphoglycerides, are the building blocks of the central nervous system. You have to get these special fats from the diet. They are essential, and you cannot make them without eating the foods containing them, so they are called *essential fatty acids.* (These are explained in more detail in Chapter 4.) Essential fatty acids are needed for the brain to work properly.

Cell membranes also need these essential fatty acids (as well as proteins) to be built properly. Cell membranes must have fluidity and flexibility to be in good shape. They get this fluidity and flexibility from polyunsaturated fats.

Overall, therefore, the body has a great need for polyunsaturated fats. That's why a diet high in polyunsaturated fats and low in saturated fat is so important for MS.

DO PEOPLE WITH MS HAVE A DEFECT IN FAT METABOLISM?

Does MS develop against a background of inborn mishandling of certain essential fatty acids? This idea was the brainchild of Professor R. H. S. Thompson of the Middlesex Hospital. This innate defect in handling fats has become known as "Thompson's anomaly."

Professor Thompson was the first to put forward the suggestion that people with MS lacked certain essential fatty acids (linoleic acid and arachidonic acid) in their cell membranes. As I have said, unsaturated fatty acids form an important constituent of the phospholipids, which are a component of cell surface membranes everywhere in the body.

Other researchers did studies to see whether Thompson was right. If he was, the surface of *all cells* in the body of someone with MS would be in some way different from those of normal people and people suffering from other neurological diseases.

One of the scientists who extended the work of Professor R. H. S. Thompson was Professor E. J. Field. He particularly studied red blood cells in people with MS and in fact devised a brilliant test that measured how fast MS red blood cells traveled in the presence of linoleic acid and arachidonic acid. This became known as the electrophoretic mobility test (see page 39).

Professor Field confirmed what had been suspected: the red blood cells in people with MS are subtly different. So are the lymphocytes (white blood cells), which should play a part in the body's immune system if they are doing their job properly. This might help explain the autoimmune aspect of MS.

One of the implications of this hypothesis is that certain people—those with anomalous cell membranes lacking in essential fatty acids—have a predisposition to MS. In other words, they are probably born with this abnormality and have the prepared soil on which MS can develop later in life. Either some "X factor" comes along to bring on the MS in an already prepared soil or the myelin is so shoddily built, at the critical time when myelin is being laid down, that in due course it simply falls apart.

The reason for nutritional therapy involving essential fatty acids is that these anomalies in cells can be corrected by eating the right foods or supplements. This is easily provable with the electrophoretic mobility test.

Reference

1. Swank, R. L., and Dugan, B. B. *The Multiple Sclerosis Diet Book.* Doubleday, 1987.

4

Fats and MS

The previous chapter explained the main thinking behind the advisability of a low fat/high polyunsaturated fat diet for anyone with MS. Before we go any further, it is important to describe the difference between the two types of fat—saturated fat and unsaturated fat.

SATURATED FATS

Saturated fats are usually hard at room temperature. Think of candles as a good example of what hard fat looks like.

Butter, hard cheeses, and the visible fat on meat are examples of saturated fat. More subtle examples of saturated fat are in such foods as manufactured cakes and cookies.

Saturated fat is not needed for any essential structures or functions of the body. Its function is to help give energy. Too much of it will be laid down in fat—the kind of fat that everyone understands: spare tires around the tummy and bulges on the thighs—in short, too much padding.

UNSATURATED AND POLYUNSATURATED FATS

Generally speaking, unsaturated fats are liquid or soft at room temperature, e.g., vegetable, seed, and fish oils. A bottle of natural sunflower seed oil or a tub of a polyunsaturated spread such as sunflower oil margarine is easy to identify as an unsaturated fat. Nowadays, the word "polyunsaturated" is written clearly on the label of such products.

Less easy to identify are the unsaturated fats hidden in foods you would not normally associate with fats at all. This list includes fish; dark green leafy vegetables; organ meats such as liver, heart, kidneys, and brains; lean meat; shellfish; and sprouting seeds.

FATTY ACIDS AND ESSENTIAL FATTY ACIDS

Fat is made from smaller components called fatty acids. In biochemical terms, fatty acids are chain-like substances, some with short chains and some with long chains. The chains are of carbon atoms with hydrogen and oxygen atoms attached. The degree of saturation depends on the extent to which the chain can absorb more hydrogen.

Unsaturated fats are capable of picking up other molecules available to them in the system. Saturated fats cannot take any more hydrogen.

- If a fatty acid has *no* double bonds, it is saturated.
- If a fatty acid has *one* double bond, it is unsaturated.
- If a fatty acid has *two or more* double bonds, it is polyunsaturated.

Figure 1 shows an example of a polyunsaturated fatty acid, linoleic acid.

The body can make some of the fatty acids it needs for growth, but it is incapable of making the essential fatty acids. Essential fatty acids are called "essential" because your body cannot make

FIGURE 1
Linoleic Acid, a Chain with Eighteen Carbon Atoms and Two Double Bonds

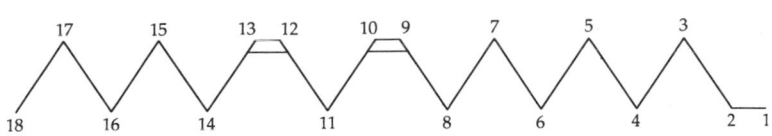

them itself. Like vitamins, essential fatty acids must be taken with the food you eat. All essential fatty acids are polyunsaturated fatty acids (PUFAs), but the reverse is not true. Not all PUFAs are essential fatty acids (EFAs). For a PUFA to act as an EFA, highly specific chemical structures are required. The polyunsaturated fatty acid must be in what is called the "cis" form to be biologically active.

Like certain vitamins, cis-linoleic acid and alpha-linolenic acid have no biological activity of their own, apart from being oxidized to provide energy. If they are to function as EFAs, they require specific biochemical transformation within the body. The exact functions of each of the fatty acids in the sequence (see Figure 2) are by no means fully known. However, it is known that unless cis-linoleic acid can be converted to gammalinolenic acid, it has no biological activity as an essential fatty acid.

"Fat" is a rather misleading word to be connected with essential fatty acids. These vital nutrients are more like proteins or vitamins. It is vital to eat them to stay healthy.

Essential fatty acids are present in every cell in your body and are vital for metabolism. These are the fats that make up a major proportion of the brain and nervous system. This type of fat is an essential part of nutrition.

The two terms "essential fatty acids" and "polyunsaturated fatty acids" can be confusing because they are not necessarily the same thing. Some doctors talk about PUFAs as if they were all essential fatty acids. For simplicity's sake, whenever PUFAs are mentioned in this book they should be taken to mean those polyunsaturated fatty acids that are also essential fatty acids.

EFAs AND MULTIPLE SCLEROSIS

The previous chapter looked in detail at why this type of fat is so important for people who have MS. To recap:

- EFAs are needed for the growth and repair of the nervous tissue.

Figure 2
How Longer Chain Fatty Acids Are Made in the Body

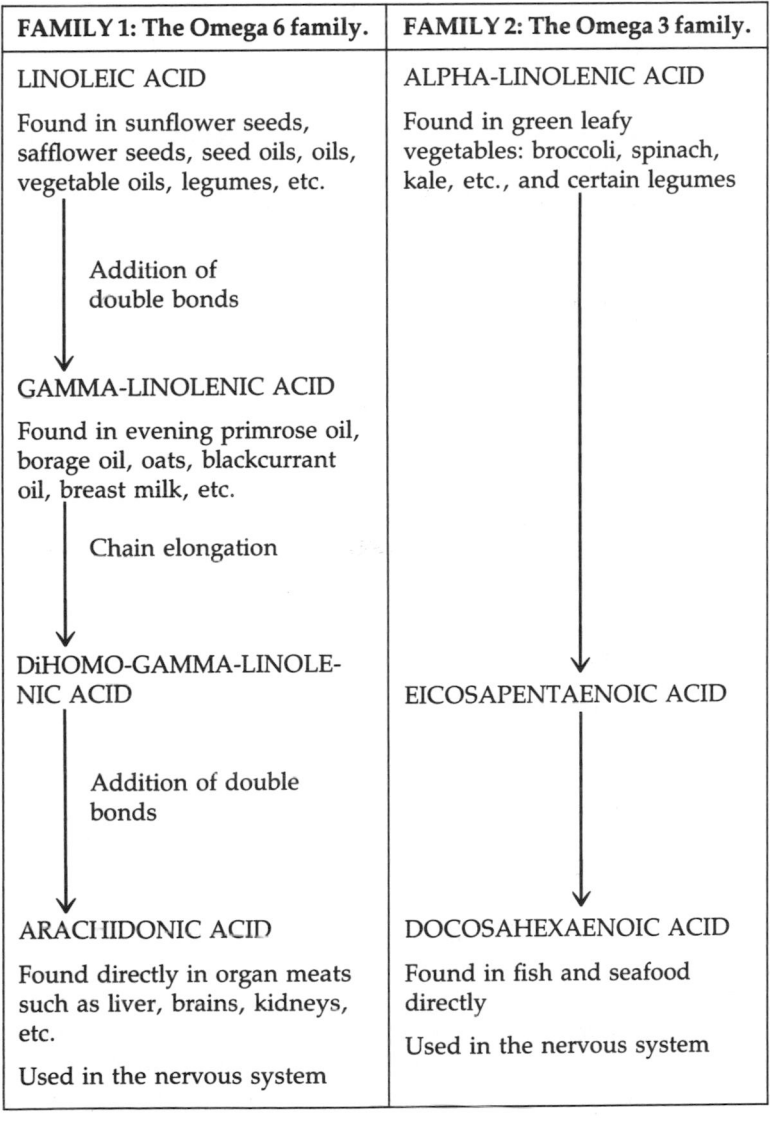

FAMILY 1: The Omega 6 family.	FAMILY 2: The Omega 3 family.
LINOLEIC ACID	ALPHA-LINOLENIC ACID
Found in sunflower seeds, safflower seeds, seed oils, oils, vegetable oils, legumes, etc.	Found in green leafy vegetables: broccoli, spinach, kale, etc., and certain legumes
Addition of double bonds	
GAMMA-LINOLENIC ACID	
Found in evening primrose oil, borage oil, oats, blackcurrant oil, breast milk, etc.	
Chain elongation	
DiHOMO-GAMMA-LINOLE-NIC ACID	EICOSAPENTAENOIC ACID
Addition of double bonds	
ARACHIDONIC ACID	DOCOSAHEXAENOIC ACID
Found directly in organ meats such as liver, brains, kidneys, etc.	Found in fish and seafood directly
Used in the nervous system	Used in the nervous system

- EFAs are needed for the maintenance of the structure of nervous tissue. This is particularly important in MS, in which the nervous system is under attack. If the body lacks these nutrients, any repair of damaged tissue is made more difficult.
- People with MS show an unusual pattern of fatty acids in their blood. With a diet rich in EFAs, this can return to normal in nine months to one year.
- Some research has shown that the white matter in the brains of people with MS is low in EFAs.
- Perhaps people with MS have an inborn inability to handle EFAs correctly.
- In people with MS, the myelin sheath, the red and white blood cells, the platelets, and the blood plasma are also deficient in EFAs, particularly linoleic acid.
- EFAs play a fundamental role in all cell membranes of the body. The fluidity and flexibility of the cell membranes depends on how much EFAs the cells have.
- The activity of lymphocytes (white blood cells) may be dependent on the state of the cell membrane. They will behave differently according to whether a cell membrane is fluid (plenty of EFAs) or rigid (not enough EFAs.) This influences the ability of certain lymphocytes to react immunologically.

THE FAMILIES OF ESSENTIAL FATTY ACIDS

There are two families of essential fatty acids. Both families are very important to the dietary management of MS.

The first family is headed by linoleic acid. Biochemists call this the Omega 6 family, and it is often referred to like this. The other family is headed by alpha-linolenic acid. Biochemists call this the Omega 3 family.

When foods containing these two families of fatty acids are eaten, the body makes them into longer chain, more biologically active unsaturated fatty acids. It is only these longer chain fatty acids that are used by the brain.

The derivatives of linoleic acid and alpha-linolenic acid are more important for the brain and nervous system than the parent fatty acids. This means that gamma-linolenic acid and arachidonic acid are more important than linoleic acid and that eicosapentaenoic and docosahexaenoic acids are more important than alpha-linolenic acid.

THE DERIVATIVES OF ESSENTIAL FATTY ACIDS

It is fine to eat the parent foods, but only a small amount of the derivatives are actually produced in this way. In any case, it is thought that people with MS may not be as efficient as other people in converting the parent essential fatty acids to their derivatives. This is an explanation for the abnormal EFA blood profile of people with MS and means it is better to eat directly the foods containing gamma-linolenic acid, arachidonic acid, eicosapentaenoic acid, and docosahexaenoic acids.

Gamma-linolenic Acid

Gamma-linolenic acid (GLA) is 50 percent more unsaturated than linoleic acid. It is not present in any of the commercially produced vegetable oils; in fact, it is quite rare. The easiest way to take it is in capsules of evening primrose oil, which contain about 9 percent GLA. It is also available in blackcurrant seed oil capsules, borage oil capsules, and oats, and GLA is now being developed from a special mold. (See Chapter 7 on evening primrose oil.) From GLA it is easy for the body to make some prostaglandins, which are vital for good health.

Arachidonic Acid

Arachidonic acid is one of the most important and effective of the essential fatty acids. It plays a vital role in the structure of healthy cells and is involved in the production of prostaglandins. It may also play a part in the regulation of the body's immune system. Liver is the best and easiest to obtain source of arachidonic acid.

FIGURE 3
The Various Ways in Which EFAs May Work in the Treatment of MS

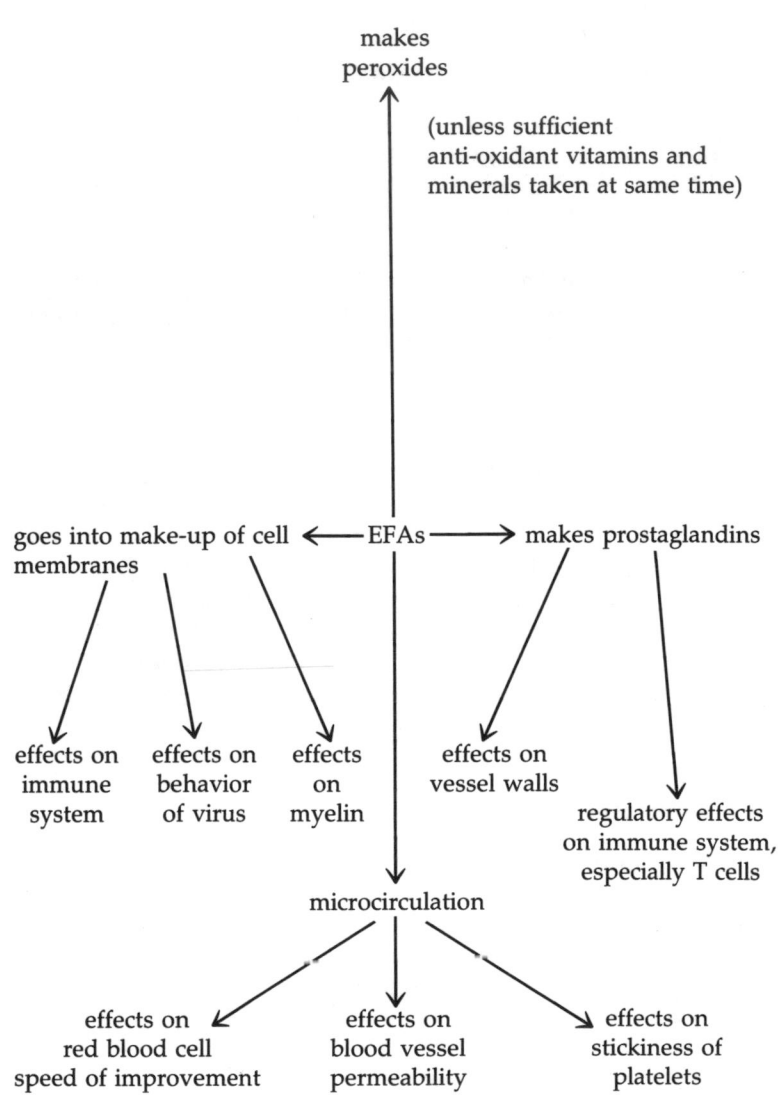

Prostaglandins

Prostaglandins may be a vital key to the MS mystery. They are manufactured from dihomo-gamma-linolenic acid and from arachidonic acid.

Prostaglandins are a newly understood class of substance. They have a hormone-like character. Like hormones, they act as regulatory substances and as messengers. Unlike hormones, which are normally produced by a gland, prostaglandins are not produced by glands. They are produced and used very locally, as and when they are needed. They are metabolized on site and used very quickly.

Prostaglandins have two particularly important functions related to MS—platelet aggregation and regulation of the immune system. The platelets are very small particles in the blood. They play a role in blood clotting. In MS, there is evidence to show that there is an abnormal "clumping together" of platelets. Prostaglandins are thought to regulate the platelet functions in the blood. Using modern testing techniques, it is now possible to show that, after a diet high in EFAs is eaten for several months, the platelet behavior in the blood becomes normal. It is thought that the prostaglandins, which are metabolized from certain EFAs, play a vital role in this.

Prostaglandins and the Immune System
The other very important function that certain prostaglandins are thought to have is regulation of the immune system. Something is certainly wrong with the immune system of people with MS.

The main function of the immune system is to eliminate invading bodies, such as bacteria and viruses, from the body. MS is called an autoimmune disease. What happens is that, for some reason, the body cannot tell the difference between itself and alien matter. In the confusion, the body attacks its own substances.

The kind of prostaglandins that regulate the immune system may be in short supply in people with MS. A shortage of the series 1 prostaglandins may possibly lead to defective lymphocytes and may increase the body's susceptibility to autoimmune damage (i.e., the body producing antibodies that act against its own tissues).

Series 1 prostaglandins may be of critical importance in regulating the function of some particular white blood cells involved in defending the body—the T lymphocytes. One type of T lymphocyte, the T suppressor cells, prevents the body from attacking itself. Research has shown that levels of T suppressor cells are very low in MS patients during a relapse. It is known that prostaglandins have the effect of dampening down lymphocytes that are capable of attacking the central nervous system. So, in short, EFAs help boost the immune system.

POSSIBLE MECHANISMS BY WHICH EFAs MAY WORK IN MS

We have now looked at all the various reasons for eating a low fat/high polyunsaturated fat diet if you have MS. The mechanisms that may be involved are summarized in Figure 3.

5

Recent Research on Nutrition and MS

There have been two recent studies on the low fat/high polyunsaturated fat diet for MS. The first was done by Professor Roy Swank of the Oregon Health Sciences University in Portland, Oregon; the second was done by the ARMS Unit at the Central Middlesex Hospital, London. Both studies had the same broad conclusion—people with MS who stick steadfastly to a low fat diet *do not get worse*, whereas people who do not stick to it *do get worse*.

THE SWANK RESEARCH

Swank is very strict indeed with the amount of saturated fat that he allows per day—15 grams total. He has noticed that if patients exceed this allowance even by a small amount of fat, they slowly get worse. This can happen to patients who had been stable on the low fat diet. Once someone does slip or cheat on the low fat diet, he or she is unlikely to get back to a stable condition. Professor Swank says:

> The addition of 8 grams (1½ teaspoons) of fat often may appear to allow stabilization of the disease but this lasts for no longer than 7 years. Then the disease becomes rapidly progressive, from which there is no recovery. . . . The chance that you can tolerate more than 15 grams of fat daily is no more, and probably less, than 4 per cent. Ninety-six per cent of patients who have exceeded their saturated fat by 10 grams or more have ended up deteriorating rapidly and suffered a high death rate. There

is a sharp increase in disability and deaths upon the addition of 8 grams or more fat to the diet.

Professor Swank noted that a saturated fat intake of 20 to 25 grams will not usually produce any apparent increased disability in a short period. A slow, silent deterioration occurs, and in a few years increased activity of the disease surfaces. To exceed this level repeatedly will result in the inability to lead an active life.

In recent years, Professor Swank has noticed that many patients were increasing their saturated fat intake without realizing it. These patients were tempted to buy new products on the supermarket shelves that advertised themselves as being "low fat" or "no fat" or "pure oils" when in fact they contained saturated fat.

Professor Swank has done research on a low fat diet far longer than anyone else. He first started his research in Montreal in 1951. Although his research does not adhere to strict scientific methods, one would be foolish to ignore his very impressive results.

Since 1951, Professor Swank has been following the cases of 150 patients with MS. He has looked at the relationship of their fat intake to the progress of disability and the number of deaths. He plotted a graph of those patients who ate less than 20 grams of fat a day, those eating 20 to 30 grams of fat a day, and those eating more than 30 grams of fat a day. By the end of the study, 21 percent of the patients eating less than 20 grams of fat a day had died, but Swank concluded that a slight increase of no more than an average of 8 grams of fat per day more than doubled the death rate to 54 percent. The patients in his study who ate the most saturated fat deteriorated the most and had the highest death rates.

For those who have stuck faithfully to Swank's low fat diet, the success has been remarkable. Swank says that 90 to 95 percent of patients who began his diet in the early stages of MS, with little or no evident disability, did not get worse during thirty-five years on the diet.

Patients who started the diet later in the course of the disease, with definite disability, did get worse, but at a much slower rate than would have been expected. In a few cases, the condition stabilized.

Professor Swank says that his diet prolongs active, productive life. Patients got stronger and remained energetic, stable, and attack-free. Old signs and symptoms may still have been there, but new ones rarely developed.

Patients who started the diet after becoming disabled noted an increased feeling of well-being. Most patients had fewer colds and stomach upsets and noted an increase in energy. There was a 95 percent reduction in the frequency of attacks, and the attacks that did occur were mild, infrequent, and brief.

Professor Swank found that patients on the low fat diet were able to work and walk longer. About 50 percent of MS patients on no specific diet who could work and walk at the beginning could not do so at the end of ten years, whereas only 25 percent of Swank's patients, all on the low fat diet, could not work or walk after ten years.

Death rates are lower too. By Swank's figures, the average death rate among people with MS on the low fat diet is two-thirds to three-quarters the normal death rate for MS sufferers.[2]

THE ARMS EFA-RICH DIET: RESULTS OF RESEARCH

Action for Research into Multiple Sclerosis (ARMS) is a self-help group for MS sufferers in the United Kingdom. All members have MS themselves, are related to someone with MS, or have a close interest in MS. The organization was founded in 1974 by a small group of people with MS who were angry that not enough was being done in the field of MS research, particularly research that might be considered unorthodox. Since then, the membership has grown to several thousand, and ARMS funds its own research, the most prominent of which has to do with MS and nutrition. ARMS also has its own research unit at a London hospital, where patients participate in therapy involving nutrition, physiotherapy, and counseling.

The main results of a three-year study conducted by ARMS were that patients who carefully followed the dietary advice did not deteriorate, whereas those who did not stick closely to the diet deteriorated significantly. The diet was devised by Michael Crawford, Professor of Nutrition at Nottingham University. All patients taking part in the study had clinically diagnosed multiple sclerosis. They were eighty-three of the three hundred and sixty people attending the ARMS Unit at the Central Middlesex Hospital in London for nutrition, physiotherapy, and counseling therapy.

The results of the three-year study were published in September 1986. For ethical reasons, there was no control group, so the research cannot be called a trial. However, as several people in the group did not comply with the dietary advice given, it was possible to compare the progress of those who stuck faithfully to the diet with that of those who did not.

The aims of the study were to improve the general health of the MS patients by nutrition and also to find out whether this nutritional management of MS worked. To see if these two aims were being achieved, Professor Crawford and his associates worked out a "nutrient scoring system" and set target levels for particular nutrients. In other words, they devised the "ideal diet."

ARMS Nutrient Target Levels

No one knows for certain to what extent MS alters the daily requirement for nutrients over and above that of a healthy person. However, it is likely that people with a chronic disease like MS do have an increased need for the nutrients involved in the conversion and protection of fatty acids. So the daily intake of certain nutrients was set above that recommended by the Department of Health and Social Security. (See Table 1.)

The Nutrient Scoring System

Points were awarded for particular nutrients. A person's score depended mostly on the consumption of each nutrient. Target levels were set for each of the nutrients.

Points were awarded for kilocalories, total fat, the ratio between polyunsaturated and saturated fat, the ratio between linoleic and alpha-linolenic acid, fiber, vitamin E, vitamin C, folate, vitamin B_{12}, vitamin B_6, and zinc. Bonus points were awarded to highlight the importance of balance in the diet. Two special groups were minerals (copper, zinc, iron, and calcium) and vitamins (vitamins A, D, and E). If all of the nutrients in each category were within the ARMS target (see Table 1), a bonus of 5 points was given. Deductions of points were made if the amount of PUFAs fell below 10 grams, as this is thought to be the minimal level. The maximal score possible was 140 points.

Results

After patients had been on the ARMS diet for six months, the mean nutrient score for women had gone up from 48 points at the start of the study to 79 points. After thirty months on the diet, the mean score was 84. For men, the mean score started at 66 points, went up to 95 points at six months, and stayed at 95 at thirty months. For both women and men, the biggest changes were made during the first six months.

In all, the total amount of fat consumed went down, the ratio between polyunsaturated and saturated fat changed in favor of polyunsaturated fats, and the intake of all nutrients went up. In women, the total number of calories consumed came down.

Neurological Results

Significant results emerge when the results are divided between people who had a high score on the nutrient scoring system and those who had low scores. The ones with high scores showed no significant differences in the Kurtzke disability scale over the three years. However, the ones with low nutrient scores got significantly worse throughout the study. The high score group had fewer and shorter relapses.

For the group as a whole, the Kurtzke disability scale showed that the mean Kurtzke score did not change significantly over the three-year study. Within the group, 68 percent either stayed the same or deteriorated slightly, while 32 percent deteriorated

TABLE 1
Recommended Nutrient Levels

Nutrients	Sex	Recommended Daily Allowance	ARMS Target
Calories	M	2,510	2,000
	F	2,150	1,800
Fiber (grams)	M	30 grams (COMA/ NACNE)	30 grams
	F	30 grams	30 grams
Calcium	M	500 mg	800 mg
(mg)	F	500 mg	800 mg
Iron (mg)	M	10 mg	16 mg
	F	12 mg	16 mg
Copper	M	1–3 mg	4 mg
(mg)	F	1–3 mg	4 mg
Zinc (mg)	M	9–12 mg	12 mg
	F	9–12 mg	12 mg
Vitamin A	M	750 μg	not more than 6,000
(μg)	F	750 μg	not more than 6,000
Vitamin D	M	up to 10 μg	up to 15 μg
(μg)	F	up to 10 μg	up to 15 μg
Thiamin	M	1.0 mg	1.7 mg
(mg)	F	0.9 mg	1.5 mg
Riboflavin	M	1.6 mg	3.3 mg
(mg)	F	1.3 mg	3.0 mg
Nicotinic	M	18 mg	25 mg
acid (mg)	F	15 mg	23 mg
Vitamin C	M	30 mg	120 mg
(mg)	F	30 mg	120 mg
Vitamin E	M	5–10 mg	12 mg
(mg)	F	5–10 mg	12 mg
Vitamin B_{12}	M	3–4 μg	30 μg
Folic acid	M	300 μg	350 μg
(μg)	F	300 μg	350 μg
Vitamin B_6	M	no RDA set	2.0 mg
(mg)	F	no RDA set	2.0 mg

to a greater extent. These figures are comparable with the results of immunosuppressive drug trials, but without the side effects from drugs.[3]

Results Using Blood Measurements of EFAs and the Electrophoretic Mobility Test
It was possible to monitor changes in the diet by measuring the EFA content of the blood. The levels of PUFAs rose with the diet.

After participants had followed the diet for a year, the red blood cell (electrophoretic) mobility increased to the normal level in 82 percent of the subjects. This level was maintained as long as the diet was followed. If the diet deteriorated for any reason, then the red blood cell mobility fell below normal.

The Effect of Diet on Red Blood Cell Membranes

Method
Forty patients were randomly selected from patients following the diet and exercise program at the ARMS Unit at the Central Middlesex Hospital. Patients were advised about the ARMS essential fatty acids diet. They were matched against a control group in terms of age and sex.

Blood samples were taken before and at three-monthly intervals after patients started the diet. Control subjects did not follow any diet but gave blood samples at the same intervals. All blood samples were coded and tested "blind"—that is, the scientists did not know to whom the blood belonged. The samples were decoded only after the results had been obtained. All samples from patients and their controls taken over one year were tested together.

Red blood cells were extracted from whole blood and measured for their membrane surface charge by use of a laser cytopherometer. The scientists involved in this study had previously found that approximately 75 percent of patients with MS have red blood cells with a low surface charge, as indicated by a slow electrophoretic mobility (EPM). This blood abnormality is seen in only a small proportion of control subjects, most of whom are smokers.

Results
Blood samples taken from patients before they started the diet showed a slow electrophoretic mobility. By six to twelve months after starting the diet, however, most patients had blood cells that gave readings in the normal range. The diet had therefore in some way "corrected" this abnormality.

In a small group of patients, exhaustive analysis of red blood cell membrane composition was carried out. Before the diet was started, most patients with MS had a low level of linoleic acid in their blood cells. However, a more unexpected finding was that these cells also contained high levels of nervonic acid, a fatty acid not normally detected in red blood cells of people who do not have MS. The scientists thought that the most probable source of the nervonic acid was the breakdown of myelin in the central nervous system.

After some time on the diet, however, linoleic acid levels were raised to normal and nervonic acid levels fell. Again, this represents a "normalization" of red blood cell properties. What is more, these changes correlated very strongly with the changes in red blood cell surface charge.

These results may mean that patients *who stick closely to the low saturated/high PUFA diet* (the ARMS diet) have less demyelination and therefore less damage. This would fit with recent findings that patients on the diet seem to have shorter and less severe relapses.[4] Professor Michael Crawford believes that the diet may work as a remission agent.

OTHER STUDIES ON FATS AND MS

The first trial that set the ball rolling was in 1973 and tested sunflower seed oil. The scientists involved were Millar, Zilkha, and others. The important conclusion was that the frequency, severity, and duration of attacks were reduced in the group who took the sunflower seed oil.[5]

In 1978, a trial was conducted by Professor David Bates and co-workers at Newcastle University.[6] They divided one hundred sixteen patients with MS into four groups. Group A was given Naudicelle capsules of evening primrose oil; group B was given capsules of olive oil; group C was given Flora polyunsaturated margarine spread made with sunflower seed oil; and group D was given a placebo spread.

When the patients' conditions were measured on a disability scale, there was no significant difference between the four groups after two years. However, the duration and severity of attacks was less in the group treated with the Flora sunflower seed oil spread. In this group, the blood linoleate levels had increased to 28 to 39 percent by the end of the trial period.

Interestingly, there was no significant elevation of linoleate in the group who were given six capsules of evening primrose oil a day. Professor Bates concluded that one had to take in enough polyunsaturates to affect the plasma levels of linoleate before there would be any effect on the severity and duration of relapses. Obviously, people were taking in more PUFAs from eating sunflower seed margarine than from taking six capsules of evening primrose oil without any additional source of PUFAs. However, at the time of this trial in Newcastle, Naudicelle capsules had orange and black shells, which contained the yellow dye tartrazine. It is now known that tartrazine will inhibit the uptake of PUFAs, and this could have reduced the effectiveness of the treatment. Evening primrose oil capsules now come in clear gelatin shells.

Sometimes this Newcastle study is quoted by people who want to prove that evening primrose oil is not effective in MS. In fact, the Newcastle study—far from showing the ineffectiveness of polyunsaturates for MS—does the opposite. It shows that someone with MS needs to take a certain amount of linoleate for it to be effective and also that this will help only certain patients.

Some years after the Newcastle study, a Canadian doctor, Robert Dworkin,[7] looked closely at the results of this Newcastle trial, but he also pooled these results together with results from two other trials, one performed jointly in London and Belfast

(Millar and others) and one done in Ontario. What Dr. Robert Dworkin found was extremely important: *patients who had very low levels of disability at the start of the trial, who took polyunsaturates, did not get worse in a two-year period.*

This was indeed a crucial discovery—the length of time that a patient had had MS made a difference to the outcome of the trials. The newly diagnosed, who were 0 to 2 on the Kurtzke disability scale at the start of the trial, were the ones who showed little change or deterioration by the end of the trial. This applied only to the groups that had been treated with PUFAs. The conclusion from this is that *treatment with PUFAs helps to stabilize MS in the recently diagnosed who have no real disability.* Dworkin's study proves these points:

- There *is* a treatment for MS.
- Early diagnosis is therefore vital so that treatment can start without delay.
- If the newly diagnosed are given polyunsaturates (PUFAs), they stand a good chance of stabilizing.

At Last PUFAs Get Taken Seriously

For the last ten years or so, many people with MS who have been taking polyunsaturates have been laughed at by the medical profession. My own view, which has always backed PUFAs, has been dismissed with derision (especially, ironically, by the MS Society in Canada!) So it gives me great pleasure to see that, at long last, some orthodox doctors are backing PUFAs—and this includes some doctors who scoffed at the whole idea some years ago.

The following is taken from *MS News*, published by the Multiple Sclerosis Society of Great Britain and Northern Ireland, Winter 1986 edition. The article is "Polyunsaturated Oils and the Treatment of MS" by Dr. Tony Smith.[8]

"Three independent carefully controlled trials have indicated that, for some patients, dietary polyunsaturated oils can have a beneficial therapeutic effect on the course of MS . . ."

Dr. Smith said that analysis of the pooled data from the three centers

> . . . gave powerful support to the concept that dietary oil treatment could help some patients with MS. This analysis confirmed that the oil shortened relapses and reduced their severity, and also indicated that, for some patients, the oils could favourably affect the overall rate of deterioration. . . . Considering that the data are derived from three independent, carefully controlled trials, the results must be taken very seriously.

Of course, more research must be done. Dr. Smith emphasized this fact and described some research concerning PUFAs currently in progress, which is being funded by the MS Society.

CONCLUSION

Even though scientists feel they must continue with scientific trials, there is nothing to keep you from taking supplements of polyunsaturates *now*. You could hedge your bets about what works best by taking *all* the PUFAs tested in the trials.

- You could use sunflower seed oil for cooking and in salad dressings.
- You could use a sunflower seed margarine as a spread.*
- You could take capsules of evening primrose oil.
- You could take capsules of fish oils (or you could take a capsule that combines evening primrose oil and fish oils, such as Efacom, distributed by Nature's Way Products).

References

2. Interim results written in *Multiple Sclerosis News Letter* by Professor Roy Swank, Department of Neurology, Oregon Health Sciences Uni-

---

* Margarines that contain whey are not suitable for anyone avoiding milk products. Some sunflower seed margarines contain no milk products.

versity, 3181 S.W. Sam Jackson Rd., Portland, OR 97201. Full results published in *The Swank Low-Fat Diet for MS* (Doubleday, 1987).

3. Research results presented at the International Symposium on Multiple Sclerosis at Charing Cross and Westminster Medical School, London, September 24–26, 1986. Published by ARMS.

4. "Long term studies on the effect of diet on the red blood cell membranes of patients with multiple sclerosis." By Dr. R. Jones and Dr. A. Preece (Bristol Royal Infirmary); Mr. L. Harbige and Professor M. Crawford (Nuffield Laboratories, Regent's Park, London), and Dr. A. Forti, ARMS Research Unit. Research results presented at the International Symposium on Multiple Sclerosis at Charing Cross and Westminster Medical School, London, September 24–26, 1986. Published by ARMS in *Symposium Summaries*.

5. Millar, J. H. D., Zilkha, K. J., Longman, M. J. S., et al. *British Medical Journal* 1:765, 1973.

6. Bates, D., Fawcett, P. R. W., Shaw, D. A., and Weightman, D. *British Medical Journal* 2:765, 1973.

7. Dworkin, R., Bates, D., Millar, J. H. D., and Paty. *Neurology* 34:1441–1445, 1984.

8. Smith, T. Polyunsaturated oils and the treatment of MS. *MS News*, Winter 1986.

6

Low Saturated Fat/High PUFA Diets

The key to these diets is not just that they cut down drastically on saturated fat, but that at the same time they considerably increase your intake of polyunsaturated fats. When Professor Swank first thought of a low fat diet for MS more than thirty-five years ago, he only emphasized cutting down on fat, without distinguishing between good and bad fats. Thanks to scientists like Professor Hugh Sinclair, however, who has done so much frontier-breaking work on essential fatty acids, people began to think of their importance.

In the 1950s Hugh Sinclair suggested that the geographical clues about the world distribution of MS could be interpreted in another way from Swank's conclusions. Instead of simply too much fat, the vital thing to a high prevalence of MS seemed to be a low ratio of essential fatty acids to nonessential fatty acids.

Hugh Sinclair is especially famous for his work on Eskimos. Eskimos have the highest fat intake of any population, yet MS is unknown among Eskimos. The dietary fat of Eskimos is extremely rich in essential fatty acids.

The most up-to-date diets take account of the research work done on essential fatty acids over the past few decades. Swank's famous low fat diet has evolved over the years to reflect the growing awareness of the importance of essential fatty acids.

With new and sophisticated testing techniques, it is now possible to get a computer printout of the fatty acid composition of the blood. Also, the recently perfected red blood cell mobility test is able to monitor the progress of patients on a specific nutritional regimen. These data allow the diets to be scientifically analyzed and scrutinized.

THE ARMS DIET—THE ESSENTIAL FATTY ACID DIET

The ARMS diet has these main features:

- Avoid animal fats like butter, lard, suet, meat drippings, cheese, cream, and whole milk.
- Choose lean meat. Trim all fat off the meat before cooking.
- Use polyunsaturated margarine and oil. (Make sure that these have not been processed and hydrogenated.)
- Eat at least three fish meals a week.
- Eat organ foods: liver is best—eat ½ lb of liver a week.
- Eat a big helping of dark green leafy vegetables every day.
- Eat some linseeds (good source of alpha-linolenic acid) or products made with linseeds every day.
- Eat a salad made of mixed raw vegetables every day with a French dressing made of polyunsaturated oil.
- Eat as much fresh food as possible rather than processed foods.
- Eat some fresh fruit every day.
- Eat whole foods rather than refined foods, particularly whole grain cereals and bread.
- Cut down on sugar and foods containing sugar.

The ARMS diet is designed to give a balance among the different food groups and to provide balanced nutrition in terms of vitamins, minerals, and trace elements. It is also high in fiber and accords perfectly with the recommendations made by nutritional organizations in recent years.

Fats and Oils

Good oils to use in cooking are sunflower seed oil, safflower seed oil, olive oil, sesame seed oil, soybean oil, cottonseed oil, and corn oil. All of these oils contain linoleic acid. Soybean oil contains some alpha-linolenic acid.

Be on your guard when you go shopping. Make sure you buy

only pure oils. Cold pressed oils available from health food shops are the purest.

Whichever oil you use, do not heat it to the point of smoking. Do not use oil more than once; throw it away after one use. Overheating and exposure to air damage the EFA activity. After you have opened the bottle, keep it in the fridge. The best way to eat these oils is unheated, i.e., in salad dressing.

Be careful about two oils that give the impression of being unsaturated but are in fact saturated fat—palm oil and coconut oil. Avoid them! They sometimes appear hidden in "nondairy products" such as ice cream.

It is easy nowadays to buy tubs of margarines that are high in polyunsaturates. Many brands state this very clearly on the lid. Always use a spread that is high in polyunsaturates. Some of these margarines can also be used in cooking instead of butter.

"Cis" and "Trans" Fatty Acids

You may have seen the word "cis" on the label of some margarine tubs. The only type of linoleic acid that can convert into biologically useful substances is cis-linoleic acid, which is found in the oil in its natural, unadulterated state.

Only cis-linoleic acid has any real value. Once linoleic acid is processed and hydrogenated, it turns into a biologically different form and behaves like saturated fat. What were originally biologically active essential fatty acids are turned into biologically inactive trans fatty acids.

You may never have heard of them, but trans fatty acids are false friends lurking in our everyday food. On the face of it, they look perfectly innocent—ordinary bottles of cooking oil, cartons of margarine, and a whole range of other things like chips and pastries. But beware! Trans fatty acids behave as if they were saturated fat. And, far from being essential fatty acids, they actually produce EFA deficiency states and compete with genuine EFAs for your body's time and attention. They elbow the real EFAs out of the action. The trans fatty acids that you eat make their way into tissues like the brain, heart, and lungs, and some scientists are sure that they change the properties of these tissues for the worse.

Unfortunately, when government and other bodies involved in the nation's nutrition examine the amount of fats people are eating, they lump together both trans and cis fatty acids, perhaps not being fully aware that trans fatty acids do no nutritional good at all. This means that the overall intake of real essential fatty acids is much lower than we have been led to believe.

It is interesting to ponder that only since the 1920s have significant amounts of trans fatty acids been added to the diet (though they have always existed in small amounts in dairy products). People who are interested in the geographical distribution and the increase in western diseases might find this worthy of more research.

Dairy Products

The fat in whole milk is almost all saturated—about 97 percent. Skimmed milk is much better and now much easier to obtain from your supermarket. Semi-skimmed milk (1% or 2%) still has some cream in it. Powdered skimmed milk is not as good as fresh skimmed milk.

Milk products with high fat should also be avoided. This means avoiding all kinds of cream, all kinds of hard cheeses, and creamy yogurts. Instead, go for low fat (or nonfat) yogurt, curd cheese, low fat cottage cheese, and other cheeses that are low or medium fat. Soft cheeses like Brie and Camembert can be eaten now and again.

Eggs are OK in moderation—three or four eggs a week. Egg white has no fat in it, and egg yolks have a mixture of saturated and unsaturated fats.

Meat

Lean meat is good for you to eat, as it is a source of arachidonic acid. Any meat you buy from the butcher or supermarket is likely to have a fair bit of fat on it. Trim this off before cooking. Obviously, the visible fat on meat is very rich in saturated fat.

Wild fowl or game such as partridge, venison, or pigeon has much less fat than intensively reared animals. However, this kind of meat is quite an acquired taste and is not as easy to get hold of as the more everyday kinds of meat. Go for lean pork, ham, beef, lamb, chicken, turkey, and rabbit. Do not eat the skin of chicken or turkey, as this is very fatty.

Organ meats—liver, kidneys, brains, sweetbreads—are particularly rich in arachidonic acid. Liver is the best source. The aim is to eat at least ½ lb (225 grams) of fresh liver a week. This can be any kind of liver. Liver and kidneys are also very good sources of some important minerals and vitamins such as vitamin B_{12}, which is needed by the nervous system. They also contain iron, zinc, folic acid, and vitamins A, B_1, B_2, and B_6. Dried or desiccated liver tablets cannot be eaten as a substitute for fresh liver; many of the nutrients are destroyed in the processing. Do not buy manufactured meat products such as Spam, luncheon meat, pâtés, pork pies, meat pies, sausages, and hamburgers.

Fish

The types of fish that are highest in the kind of essential fatty acids you need are shellfish and oily fish such as mackerel, herring, kippers, whitebait, tuna, crab, lobster, sardines, mussels, cod roe, sprats, squid, prawns, and shrimp. These are rich in docosahexaenoic acid, which is an essential nutrient for the brain.

White fish such as cod, flounder, and haddock or freshwater fish like salmon and trout are also fine. Fresh fish is best; frozen is second best. Canned fish (e.g., sardines, tuna) is very much third best. The oil in canned fish should be drained off. Fish can be cooked any way you like, except in butter and of course cream. Fish deep-fried at the fast food store is suspect because you don't know what oils were used. Usually the oils are hydrogenated, over-heated, and used over and over again, which means that the fish (and french fries) will be laden with saturated fat.

Vegetarians

It is not possible to follow the ARMS essential fatty acids diet perfectly and be a vegetarian, as the meat and fish are very important. It would be possible, however, to work out a modified version of the diet by replacing the meat and fish with legumes and nuts, though these do not provide the same essential fatty acids as meat.

Fruits and Vegetables

Eat plenty of fresh fruits and vegetables. All vegetables are good, but the greener they are the better, as they are an excellent source of alpha-linolenic acid and also vitamin E. Choose spinach, broccoli, kale, green pepper, parsley, and green beans. Aim to eat a large helping of one or two of these vegetables every day. Sprouted beans and grains have a lot of alpha-linolenic acid as well. Frozen fruits and vegetables are not as good as fresh ones.

At lunchtime, make it a habit to eat a raw mixed salad, with a French dressing made with a linoleic acid–rich oil. Include the colored vegetables: tomatoes, carrots, beets, red peppers, and red cabbage.

As well as being rich in minerals, fruits and vegetables are the best source of vitamin C and vitamin E. These vitamins protect the essential fatty acids from damage by the air (oxidation).

Nuts and Seeds

Nuts and seeds are a good source of essential fatty acids, as well as vitamins and trace elements. Remember that the oils richest in linoleic acid and alpha-linolenic acid are pressed from seeds.

You can eat nuts and seeds as snacks on their own or in salads, in bread, or on breakfast cereals. Choose from sunflower seeds, pumpkin seeds, sesame seeds, almonds, brazil nuts, hazelnuts, walnuts, and chestnuts.

Linseeds are the best source of alpha-linolenic acid. The actual linseeds are available from health food stores or seed sellers.

You may also be able to buy products that are split linseeds. These are more palatable than linseeds and can be sprinkled on breakfast cereals.

Nut oils are OK as long as they do not contain butter or other animal fats. Make sure that the products are pure and natural and are not hydrogenated.

Cereals

Unrefined cereals and whole grain bread are better than refined cereals and white bread. Whole grains contain the germ, and it is in the germ that essential fatty acids, vitamins, minerals, and trace elements can be found. The fiber content of whole cereals is much greater because the husk has not been removed. This provides bulk and helps bowel function. Whole wheat pastas and brown rice are also fine.

The ARMS diet recommends extra bran so that the roughage content of the overall diet is high. Constipation is a common complaint in people with MS, and bran does help prevent and relieve this. ARMS suggests starting off with one tablespoon of bran a day, spread over the whole day. This can be increased gradually to a maximum of about three tablespoons. Bran can be added to flour for cooking, or it can be sprinkled on breakfast cereals, stewed fruit, yogurt, soups and stews, etc. If you do take bran, make sure that you are drinking a lot of fluid because the action of bran is to bind to fluid in the bowel.

Many breakfast cereals are now made of unrefined cereals, and some also contain bran. Remember to use skimmed milk with your breakfast cereals.

Cakes, cookies, and pastries are danger areas if you buy them, as they are high in both saturated fats and sugar. If you can bake at home, use whole grain flour and polyunsaturated margarine to make your own cakes and pastries.

Legumes

Legumes include peas, beans, lentils, etc. The fat content of legumes is low, but what fat is there is polyunsaturated. Legumes have many uses in cooking. They are a good source of protein, as well as of alpha-linolenic acid and vitamin C.

Sugar

The ARMS nutritionists have found that many people with MS lose their appetite, do not eat much, and tend to use convenience foods. This means that they lack needed nutrients. The problem with eating foods laden with sugar is that they fill you up without giving you much nutritional benefit. For that reason, it is best to avoid sugar and sugary foods.

Recipes and Menus

The ARMS nutritionists have come up with a variety of recipe leaflets on liver, fish, beans, legumes, and whole grain flour recipes. They are now in a book called *Multiple Sclerosis—Healthy Means to Help in the Management of MS,* by Geraldine Fitzgerald and Fenella Briscol (Thorsons, 1988). The diet is explained in *Why a Diet Rich in Essential Fatty Acids* (ARMS, 4a Chapel Hill, Stansted, Essex CM24 8AG, England).

For recipe leaflets, write to:

ARMS
4a Chapel Hill
Stansted
Essex CM24 8AG, England

THE SWANK LOW-FAT DIET

Full details on the Swank diet can be found in the new edition of Professor Swank's book, *The Swank Low-Fat Diet for MS,* published by Doubleday. Over the years, Swank's diet has evolved to take account of new research that shows the importance of essential fatty acids. So, although his diet is still called the "Swank low fat diet," it should really be called the "Swank low saturated fat/high unsaturated fat diet."

In a nutshell, the Swank diet has the following guidelines:

- Oils containing essential fatty acids must be included in the quantity of at least 20 grams (four teaspoons) a day. Working, walking people could increase this to eight teaspoons, and very active people could take ten teaspoons.
- All dairy products and all processed foods containing hidden fat are excluded.
- Fat in meat, poultry, liver, and eggs must be kept to a minimum. The maximal saturated fat allowed is 3 teaspoons a day. *No red meat at all* should be eaten during the first year.

Foods Containing Essential Fatty Acids

- Sunflower seed oil, safflower seed oil, soybean oil, corn oil, linseed oil, cod liver oil, oil of evening primrose
- Polyunsaturated margarines
- Tuna fish, salmon, sardines, herring, mackerel
- Sunflower seeds, sesame seeds, peanuts (and peanut butter as long as it is not hydrogenated), almonds, cashew nuts
- Dark green leafy vegetables, such as spinach

Foods Allowed in Any Quantity

These foods contain no or very little saturated fat:

- eggs, whites only
- white fish, any kind
- shellfish, any kind
- breast of poultry with skin removed
- skimmed milk
- low fat cottage cheese
- low fat yogurt
- 99 percent fat-free cheese
- clear soups, beef or chicken broth, bouillon, consommé
- whole grain bread
- matzos
- whole grain cereals
- rice

- pasta
- cornmeal
- all fresh fruits
- all fresh vegetables (cook vegetables with steamer or eat raw)
- frozen or canned vegetables without butter
- jam, marmalade
- honey
- sugar, molasses, corn syrup, maple syrup
- jelly
- tea, coffee
- carbonated drinks
- alcoholic drinks in moderation

Moderately Allowed Saturated Fat Foods

The maximal saturated fat allowed per day is 3 teaspoons. The largest single source of fat in our diet is meat. Table 2 gives the fat content of various meats.

Forbidden Foods

- Whole milk, cream, butter, sour cream, ice cream, natural and processed cheese of any kind, all imitation dairy products (often contain palm oil, which is saturated fat)
- All hard margarines, shortening, lard, chocolate, cocoa butter, coconut, coconut and palm oils
- All packaged commercial mixes for cakes and cookies; potato chips, party-type snacks; all commercially prepared pies, cakes, pastries, doughnuts, and cookies
- All processed meat and poultry, luncheon meat, salami, frankfurters, sausages, canned meat products
- Canned foods that contain cream, meat, or dairy products

General Guidelines for the Swank Diet

Ideally, eat fresh foods. If you buy any canned or packaged foods, read the label carefully. If any product does not specify the kind of vegetable oil used, avoid it.

TABLE 2:
Fat Content of Food

Food	Amount Equal to One Teaspoon of Fat
Eggs	1 whole
Chicken gizzards	3 oz (90 g)
Chicken livers	3 oz (90 g)
Heart: calf's, beef	3 oz (90 g)
Kidney: pork, veal, lamb	3 oz (90 g)
Leg of lamb	3 oz (90 g)
Liver: beef, calf, pork	3 oz (90 g)
Tongue: calf	3 oz (90 g)
Beef, lean	2 oz (60 g)
Chicken and turkey, dark meat, skin removed	2 oz (60 g)
Chicken and turkey hearts	2 oz (60 g)
Heart: lamb	2 oz (60 g)
Ham, lean	2 oz (60 g)
Kidney: beef	2 oz (60 g)
Lamb: rib, loin, shoulder	2 oz (60 g)
Pheasant, skin removed	2 oz (60 g)
Pork, lean	2 oz (60 g)
Rabbit	2 oz (60 g)
Tongue: beef	2 oz (60 g)
Veal	2 oz (60 g)
Bacon	1 oz (30 g)
Duck	1 oz (30 g)

Weigh food after it has been cooked, not before.

Use only whole grain products, e.g., whole grain bread, brown rice, or whole wheat spaghetti.

Although this is not a vegetarian diet, most protein should be taken from foods other than red meat. At least five days a week, you should get your protein from eggs, fish, seafood, skinned chicken, or turkey breast. Fish contains as much protein and amino acids as meat and is an important part of this diet.

The fat and oil intake should be distributed over the course of the day. Eat three or four meals of about the same size, rather than snacks here and there and a heavy meal at the end of the day.

When eating out, avoid creamed foods, gravies, and sauces. Avoid fried foods, including french fries. Avoid foods cooked in butter and cream. Avoid desserts, except fruit salad.

Chinese and Japanese food is generally low in saturated fat and high in unsaturated fat, except spare ribs, duck, and deep-fried dishes.

If you are asked out to a dinner party, it is wise to warn your hostess in advance about your diet.

Lifestyle

Professor Swank publishes a monthly newsletter that goes into various aspects of living, such as advice about what to do in hot weather. He is particularly insistent that his low fat diet should be combined with adequate rest. Physical and mental fatigue must be avoided. Patients are instructed to rest a minimum of one hour a day, ideally lying down after lunch.

Professor Swank's newsletter is obtainable from:

Department of Neurology
Oregon Health Sciences University
3181 S.W. Sam Jackson Park Road
Portland, OR 97201

7

Supplements 1: Evening Primrose Oil and Fish Oils

WHY TAKE SUPPLEMENTS?

The main reason for taking supplements is that you are deficient in certain nutrients and by taking supplements you will correct the deficiency. Many people with MS are thought to have problems with absorbing certain nutrients. Another good reason for taking all of the supplements described here is because they *boost the immune system.*

Not everybody agrees that you need to take supplements. ARMS, for example, in its book on the ARMS EFA diet, says: "Supplements in the form of vitamins, minerals and oils should not be necessary. The 'Essential Fatty Acid Diet,' when followed carefully, will provide adequate amounts of all the nutrients."

The other reason that Professor Crawford is against supplements is that he is trying to encourage people to eat a diet of optimal nutrition, and he fears that taking supplements will make people eat less nutritious food. He says, "The basic principle is to meet targets set for different fatty acids using *food* rather than pills and supplements. Experience tells us that people who rely on supplements tend to ignore food, which means the nutrients not covered by the supplement suffer." I do not share the view of ARMS on supplements and will explain why I think that they are very important.

First, the key phrase about the ARMS diet is "when followed carefully." Recent results of a three-year study conducted by ARMS showed that about a third of people with MS who were given dietary advice did *not* follow it. These were described in the results as "noncompliers" and were the ones who got worse.

Although in theory it might be hoped that people would stick to a healthy diet for their own good, the evidence does not back this up. It is notoriously difficult to change one's eating habits dramatically. It is sometimes possible to do this for a short time if one is very highly motivated, but it is hard to keep it up. Again, the results of the ARMS study showed that people were most eager to improve their nutrition during the first six months, but, after that, improvements leveled off, even though there was still room for improvement. Supplements seem to be absolutely vital for the people who are simply *not* going to stick to a good diet, however hard you try to persuade them.

There are other reasons why everyone with MS would do well to take supplements, not just the "noncompliers" on the diet. Supplements such as evening primrose oil contain gamma-linolenic acid (GLA), which one cannot get from any commonly available food. It is possible for the body to make gamma-linolenic from linoleic acid, but this conversion step is somewhat blocked in people who have MS and in some other people, too.

The derivatives of GLA are particularly important, as it is from GLA that series 1 prostaglandins are produced. These are described in more detail later in this chapter.

The emphasis of the ARMS essential fatty acid diet is very much to make arachidonic acid, and that is why liver is promoted so strongly on the ARMS diet. However, a derivative of arachidonic acid, series 2 prostaglandins, may not be as good for you as the series 1 prostaglandins, which are manufactured easily from evening primrose oil but with more difficulty from foods containing linoleic acid.

Another good reason for taking supplements is that the nutrient target levels set by the ARMS diet (see page 38) are above the recommended daily allowances, although not by a great deal. There is therefore a case to be made for taking certain vitamins and minerals in far higher amounts than those targeted in the ARMS diet. Taking supplements is the only way to get these larger amounts of vitamins and minerals. This will be discussed in detail in Chapter 8 on vitamin and mineral supplements.

EVENING PRIMROSE OIL

The oil comes from the evening primrose plant (Figure 4). In recent years, this plant has gone through a metamorphosis. It used to be a humble wild flower growing alongside roadsides and railway tracks or on sand dunes. Now it is a crop that farmers cultivate and harvest on a growing scale in many countries of the world. The passage of the evening primrose from wild flower to cash crop is largely because of the medicinal potential of its oil.

There are many different types of evening primrose plant. Usually, the petals are a primrose-like yellow, and the flowers open only in the evenings. Strangely enough, the plant is not one of the primrose family at all but belongs to the rosebay willow herb family.

In 1949, the seeds of the evening primrose plant were analyzed using modern techniques. They were found to contain a high percentage of linoleic acid, plus the very rare gamma-linolenic acid. GLA is much more biologically active than linoleic acid.

Other Sources of GLA

Recently, other sources of GLA have been found and developed into commercial products. These include blackcurrant oil and borage oil and GLA made from a special mold. However, people with MS should be cautious about trying these new GLA sources. Both blackcurrant and borage oils have unusual fatty acids, which are not present in evening primrose oil and which may interfere with the action of GLA. So, in spite of their higher GLA levels, these oils may be less effective.

Evening Primrose Oil and Multiple Sclerosis

Thanks to the work of scientists like Professor R. H. S. Thompson, Professor Roy Swank, and Professor Hugh Sinclair, doctors working in the field of multiple sclerosis thought that the link between unsaturated fats and multiple sclerosis was worth in-

FIGURE 4
The Evening Primrose Plant (*Oenothera biennis*)

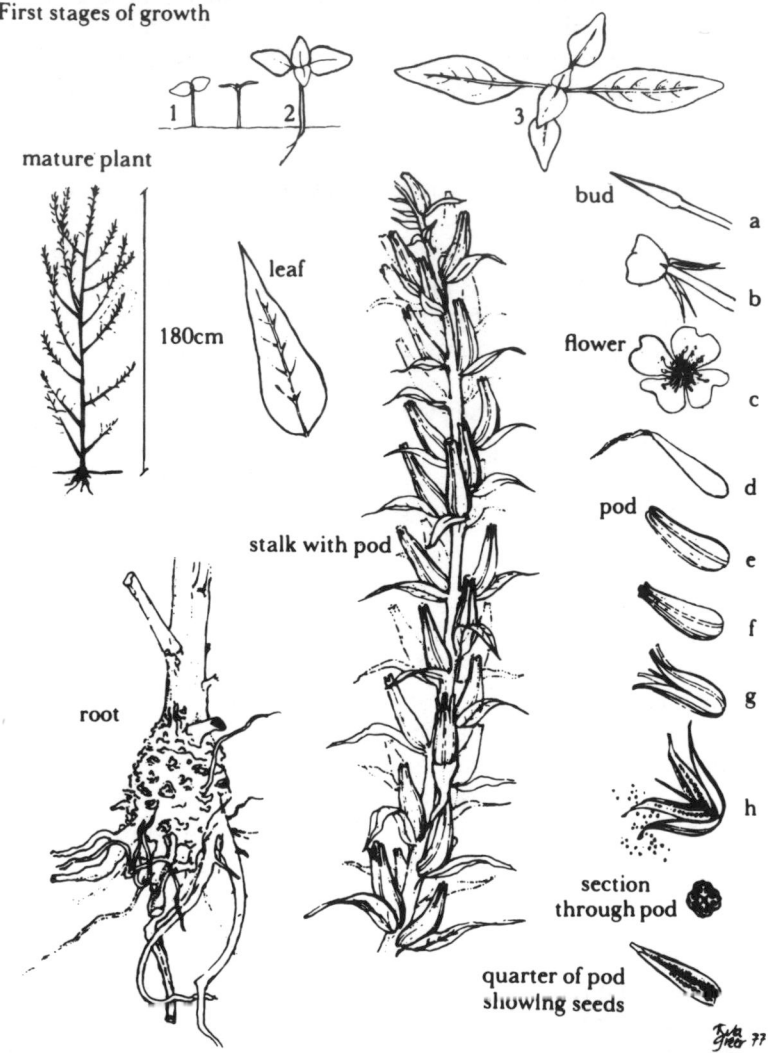

The drawings at top (1–3) show young plants with two, four, and six leaves. The stages of development of flower, pod, and seeds are shown on the right. *By kind permission of Rita Greer.*

vestigating further. The first big trial concerning linoleic acid and MS was done in 1973 by Dr. J. H. D. Millar of Belfast, Dr. K. J. Zilkha of the National Hospital in London, and others. They found that linoleic acid, in the form of sunflower seed oil, given to patients with MS reduced the frequency and severity of relapses.

After that, sunflower seed oil in various forms became all the rage with MS patients. They drank it neat; they took it in emulsions; they mixed it with orange juice. Many of them didn't like it.

At this time, evening primrose oil capsules were already being manufactured by one company only, Bio-Oil Research Ltd., of Cheshire, England. It was Bio-Oil's director, John Williams, who was the first to see the potential of evening primrose oil, originally for heart disease. When the results of the sunflower seed oil trial were published in the *British Medical Journal* in 1973, John Williams had a brainstorm. If sunflower seed oil helped MS a little, then, surely, evening primrose oil, being that much more biologically active, might help even more.

At around the same time, Professor E. J. Field was doing some very important research on essential fatty acids and MS. He started this research while Director of the Medical Research Council's Demyelinating Diseases Unit in Newcastle and later carried on with the research at the Newcastle University, funded by ARMS (at that time the Multiple Sclerosis Action Group). It was at this time that I first met Professor Field and was advised by him to start taking Naudicelle immediately.

Professor Field tested evening primrose oil on the red blood cells of people with MS. The results of the blood tests proved that the gamma-linolenic acid (GLA) in evening primrose oil was much better than linoleic acid in correcting the defects found in the blood of MS patients.

I was one of the MS patients whose blood was tested by Professor Field. After almost a year of taking evening primrose oil capsules, my EFA blood abnormalities were corrected. I was not on any particular diet at the time.

Why Evening Primrose Oil Is Better than Linoleic Acid

It has already been established that essential fatty acids belonging to the linoleic acid family (Omega 6) are vital for people with MS. The main reason that evening primrose oil is better than linoleic acid is that the conversion in the body from linoleic acid (step 1) to the next stage (step 2) is inefficient (Figure 5). Evening primrose oil, which is rich in gamma-linolenic acid, cuts out this problem altogether. After step 2, there are no problems in converting essential fatty acids into their derivative, in this case series 1 prostaglandins. Evening primrose oil starts at step 2.

There are a number of reasons why the conversion of linoleic acid to alpha-linolenic acid is inefficient, not just in people with MS but in others too. This particular stage of the metabolic pathway is fraught with possible roadblocks, or blocking agents.

Blocking Agents

These are the most common blocking agents:

- foods rich in saturated fat
- foods rich in cholesterol

FIGURE 5
The Normal Metabolic Pathway of Linoleic Acid

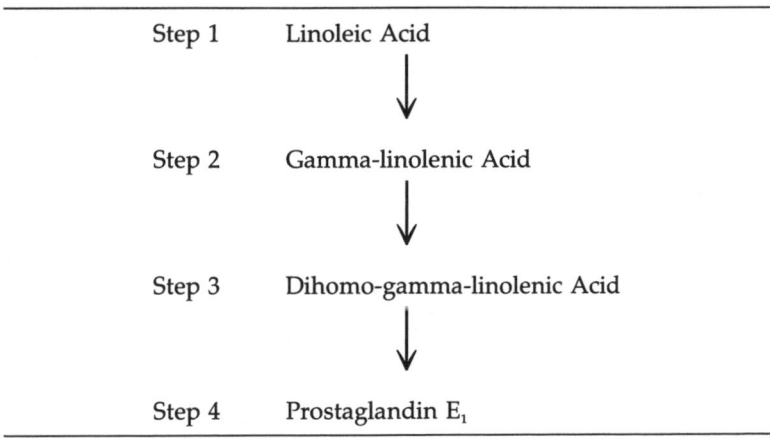

Step 1	Linoleic Acid
Step 2	Gamma-linolenic Acid
Step 3	Dihomo-gamma-linolenic Acid
Step 4	Prostaglandin E_1

- foods rich in trans fatty acids
- alcohol in moderate to large amounts
- zinc deficiencies
- the stress hormone cortisol, rampant in situations of "helplessness and hopelessness"
- viral infections
- radiation
- cancer
- ageing
- diabetes

With this information, the metabolic pathway of linoleic acid takes on a different picture (Figure 6).

Co-Factors

As can be seen from Figure 6, the process of chain elongation needs certain vitamins, minerals, and trace elements (see next chapter). The important co-factors between step 1—linoleic acid and step 2—gamma-linolenic acid are the enzyme delta 6-desaturase, vitamin B_6, biotin, zinc, and magnesium.

GLA and Prostaglandins

Evening primrose oil has an enormous head start on linoleic acid because it begins its journey at step 2, GLA, and never has to get over the obstacles in the path between step 1 and step 2. GLA, or gamma-linolenic acid, is not of great importance on its own, but it is a precursor of something that is vitally important— the series 1 prostaglandins.

The GLA in evening primrose oil will convert easily into series 1 prostaglandins. This GLA takes a different route from foods containing arachidonic acid (e.g., liver), which go on to make series 2 prostaglandins (Figure 7). There is some disagreement among scientists as to whether the EFAs eaten should favor arachidonic acid (as in the ARMS diet) or series 1 prostaglandins (taking evening primrose oil). In this debate, I back those sci-

FIGURE 6
The Bumpy Metabolic Road of Cis-Linoleic Acid

Step 1   CIS-LINOLEIC ACID
↓

Enzyme delta 6-desaturase
needed to get to step 2
↓

Helped by
zinc, magnesium, vitamin B_6, biotin
↓

BLOCKED BY SATURATED FATS

BLOCKED BY CHOLESTEROL

BLOCKED BY TRANS FATTY ACIDS

BLOCKED BY TOO MUCH ALCOHOL

BLOCKED BY TOO LITTLE ZINC

BLOCKED BY TOO MUCH CORTISOL

BLOCKED BY VIRAL INFECTIONS

BLOCKED BY TOO MUCH SUGAR

BLOCKED BY CHEMICAL CARCINOGENS

BLOCKED BY IONIZING RADIATION

BLOCKED BY AGEING
↓

Step 2   GAMMA-LINOLENIC ACID
(Evening primrose oil starts here)
↓

Step 3   DiHOMO-GAMMA-LINOLENIC ACID
↓

Helped by vitamin C, vitamin B_3 (nicotinic
acid)
↓

Step 4   PROSTAGLANDIN E_1

entists who favor taking evening primrose oil. It is fair to say that there is no hard and fast evidence to back either approach.

Prostaglandins in general are vital cell regulators. They control every cell and every organ in your body on a second-by-second basis. The nearest substances to them are hormones, which also have important messenger roles. Prostaglandins aren't like hormones, however, which zip around all over the place. Prostaglandins are much more local. They're a bit like friendly neighborhood hormones, regulating everything only on their home patch.

Each prostaglandin has a very specific effect in each tissue. Generally, prostaglandins help to control what each and every cell is doing, and they regulate the activity of certain key enzymes. Prostaglandins have a very short life span. Most prostaglandins are removed from the blood during a single passage through the lungs.

FIGURE 7
The Precursors to Prostaglandins 1 and 2

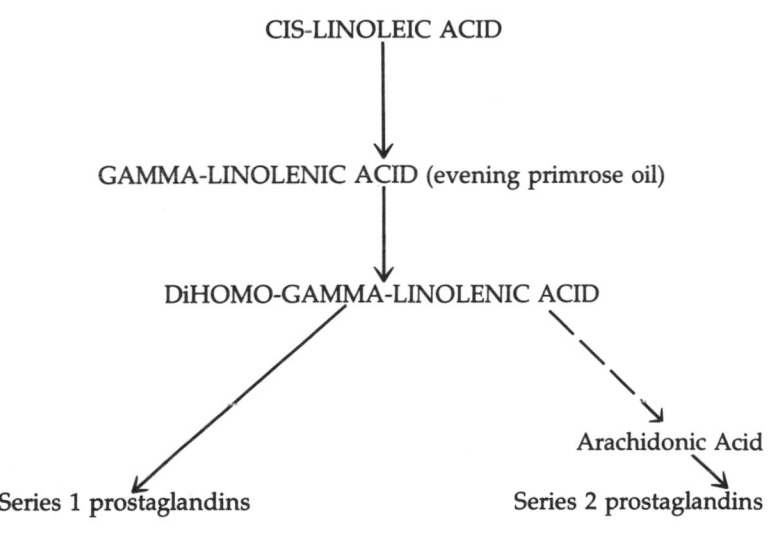

CIS-LINOLEIC ACID

GAMMA-LINOLENIC ACID (evening primrose oil)

DiHOMO-GAMMA-LINOLENIC ACID

Arachidonic Acid

Series 1 prostaglandins

Series 2 prostaglandins

Types of Prostaglandins

There are three series of prostaglandins—PG1, PG2, and PG3. Each of these has a different chemical structure, and just to make things more complicated, within each series there are many types of PGs, such as A, B, D, E, and F. In all, there are at least thirty prostaglandins.

In humans, the three series of prostaglandins are each derived from a different fatty acid. Series 1 and 2 both come from the linoleic acid family. Series 3 PGs are from eicosapentaenoic acid, a member of the alpha-linolenic acid family, and are most commonly found in oily seafoods. Evening primrose oil, whose active ingredient is gamma-linolenic acid, is a precursor of series 1 PGs.

Prostaglandins 1 (PGE$_1$)

Of all the prostaglandins researched so far, PGE$_1$ seems to have the most highly desirable qualities. In brief, these are just some of the good things for which it is responsible:

- dilation of blood vessels
- lowering of arterial pressure
- inhibition of thrombosis
- inhibition of cholesterol synthesis
- inhibition of inflammation
- activation of defective T lymphocytes
- inhibition of platelet aggregation

It's worth stressing again that PGE$_1$ is derived from alpha-linolenic acid, which is the active ingredient of evening primrose oil. This particular prostaglandin is *not* derived from eating lean meat, liver, or any of the foods rich in arachidonic acid. In fact, arachidonic acid has as its derivative the series 2 prostaglandins, which, by comparison with PG1, are more involved in inflammatory processes. My own opinion is that, because evening primrose oil goes on to make series 1 prostaglandin, it should be taken as a supplement in addition to following a low fat/high polyunsaturated fat diet.

How Evening Primrose Oil Might Be Working in MS

It Stimulates the T Lymphocytes (i.e., it boosts the immune system).
Prostaglandin E_1 stimulates the normal function of T suppressor lymphocytes. These are white blood cells that keep the other parts of the immune system under control and that make sure that the body's defenses attack foreign materials and not the body's own tissues. When T suppressor cells are defective, autoimmune damage frequently occurs. Research has shown that T suppressor cells are very low in MS patients during a relapse, and prostaglandin E_1 may help prevent this. It is known that PGE_1 has the effect of dampening down the B lymphocytes, which are capable of attacking the central nervous system.

It Keeps the Platelets from Clumping Together.
In MS, there is evidence to show that the platelets clump together in an abnormal way. The platelets are the small plate-like particles in the blood that help the blood clot. PGE_1 regulates the platelets and keeps them from bunching up and sticking to each other and to blood vessel walls.

It Makes Faulty Red Blood Cells Return to Normal.
In MS, red blood cells are not only very low in essential fatty acids but also much bigger than they ought to be, and they have a poor ability to regulate the passage of fluids through cell membranes. Evening primrose oil can correct this defect within a matter of months.

Evening primrose oil has also been shown to correct the defect in the mobility of red blood cells. Electrophoretic mobility tests have shown that the red blood cells of people with MS move more slowly than those of healthy people. After several months of evening primrose oil supplements, these red blood cells have been shown to behave normally.

In a recent follow-up study of MS patients on long-term treatment with evening primrose oil (Naudicelle) who were also following a diet low in saturated fat, it was found that the mobility of the red blood cells returned to normal. The most responsive patients were those who had experienced frequent relapses.

It Strengthens Blood Vessel Walls.
Prostaglandin E_1 is known to strengthen blood vessel walls. This is particularly important in MS. There is growing evidence that, in the microcirculation of people with MS, the blood vessel walls are breached so that blood—which is toxic to nerve tissue— seeps into the brain. When the blood vessel walls are strengthened, they are also better able to keep platelets and cholesterol from clumping together and sticking to them.

Some people believe that partly digested food is able to get through the intestinal walls in people with MS which may be a factor in food allergies. PGE_1 may help here too.

It Possibly Acts as an Anti-Viral Agent.
When human cells become transformed by viruses, they always lose the ability to convert linoleic acid to gamma-linolenic acid, and so can't make PGE_1. This may make the transformed cells resistant to attack by the body's natural defenses, the immune system. Evening primrose oil gets over this problem by its ability to convert easily into PGE_1. PGE_1 may restore the cells' normal susceptibility to the body's immune system.

It Affects the Nervous System.
Prostaglandin E_1 has effects on nerve conduction and on the action of nerves. These effects can produce profound changes in the workings of both the central nervous system and the peripheral nervous system. PGE_1 has strong regulating effects on the release of neurotransmitters at nerve endings and also on the post-synaptic actions of the released transmitters.

It Maintains a Healthy Balance Between the Series 1 and 2 Prostaglandins.
If the body is very low in essential fatty acids, there is a sharp rise in the series 2 PGs, which are made from arachidonic acid. A high level of the series 2 PGs is a feature of various inflammatory disorders, such as rheumatoid arthritis and probably

multiple sclerosis. It has recently been shown that the cerebrospinal fluid from MS patients contains high levels of PGF_2a.

Once you increase the amount of essential fatty acids in the diet, PGE_1 is back on the scene. Enough PGE_1 means that there is a healthy balance in the amount of series 1 and 2 prostaglandins being produced.

Evening primrose oil also makes it more likely that PGE_1 will be produced rather than PG_2. At the junction where the road forks at dihomo-gamma-linolenic acid, evening primrose oil persuades the traveler to follow the route toward PGE_1 instead of taking the route toward arachidonic acid and the series 2 PGs (see Figure 8).

Reported Benefits of Evening Primrose Oil for People with MS

Many of the reported benefits of evening primrose oil are anecdotal—numerous personal stories told either by letter or by word of mouth. Obviously, this is not scientific evidence and will not be good enough for hard scientists. This wealth of anecdotal evidence, however, will be heartening to people who actually have MS.

During 1979, a survey was carried out by Bio-Oil Research Ltd. to assess the views of MS patients taking Naudicelle as a dietary supplement. Of four hundred eighty MS sufferers taking part in the survey, 65 percent felt there was some improvement in their condition. Of these, 43 percent said there had been a stabilization of their condition (they had gotten neither better nor worse), 22 percent said there had been fewer and less severe attacks, 20 percent said certain symptoms had been alleviated, 13 percent reported an improvement in general health, and 2 percent reported further beneficial side effects. The overall results look like this:

Some improvement	65%
No change	22%
Deteriorated	10%
Don't know	3%

FIGURE 8
How Evening Primrose Oil Favors the PGE$_1$ Route

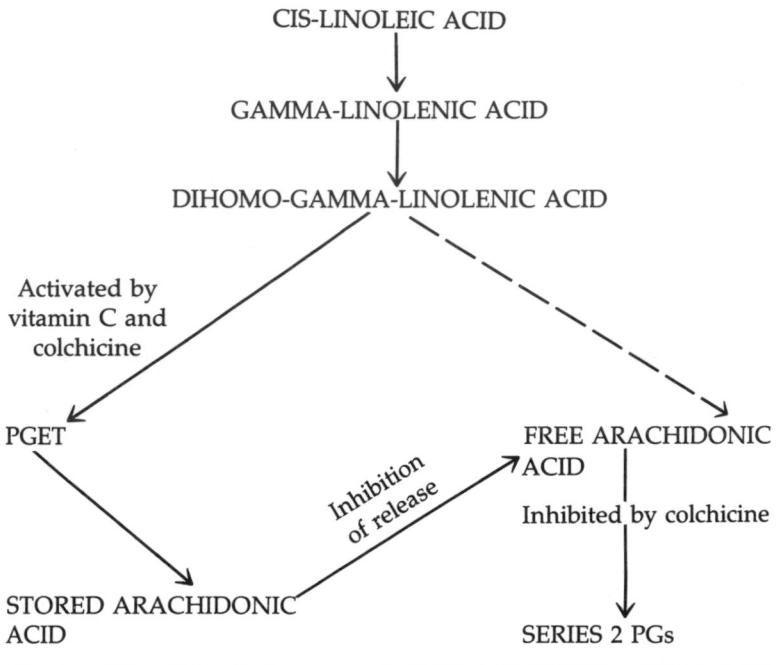

Improvements

People in the "some improvement" category mentioned the following benefits:

- increased mobility
- increased walking ability
- reduced spasm or tremor
- improved bladder function
- improved eyesight
- improved condition of hair and skin
- relief of constipation
- improvement in wound healing

- regain to correct weight
- normalization of heavy periods

Note: The "improved" group contained a significantly higher proportion of MS patients who had been diagnosed within the preceding four years.

The ARMS Survey
In 1977, ARMS sent out a questionnaire to all of its members to find out what effect Naudicelle was having on them. They were also asked to get an opinion from their own physician as to their condition since beginning to take the capsules. These are the results of the 177 completed questionnaires returned:

Improved	127
No change	33
Worse	17

Of the 127 in the "improved" category, there were 59 testimonials from physicians supporting this assessment. (Not everybody who filled in the questionnaire bothered to see a doctor.) Even though this survey has no scientific standing and all of the answers are based only on the subjective opinions of the MS sufferers who filled in the questionnaire, the results are nevertheless extremely encouraging.

ARMS members were also asked how long they had been taking Naudicelle. The answers showed that improvements increased when they had been taking the capsules for more than four months. Beneficial effects appeared as follows:

DURATION OF CAPSULE USE	PERCENTAGE REPORTING BENEFICIAL EFFECTS
Under 4 months	35%
4 months to 1 year	73%
1 to 2 years	73%
2 to 3 years	82%

At the time of the survey, very few members had been on Naudicelle for longer than three years.

Of the people who returned the completed questionnaires, 141 were also on some kind of special diet. The people who were on a low saturated fat diet had better results with evening primrose oil.

Clinical Trials of Evening Primrose Oil and MS

Two clinical trials involving evening primrose oil took place in Newcastle in 1978, conducted by Professor David Bates and others. (*Note:* Both studies took place before Efamol or other brands were available on the market.)

The researchers divided one hundred and sixteen people with MS into four groups. One group was given evening primrose oil, Naudicelle, six capsules a day; one group was given olive oil in capsules; one group was given Flora margarine to eat as a spread; one group was given another spread. (No one knew what they were taking.) At the end of the two years, there was no significant difference among the groups, as measured by the Kurtzke disability scale.

Of all the groups, those who did best were the ones who took the sunflower seed oil spread Flora. The duration and severity of their attacks were less. In this group, the amount of linoleate in their blood went up from 28 percent before the trial started to 39 percent at the end of the trial.

Professor Bates came to the conclusion that polyunsaturates have to be taken in amounts sufficient to affect plasma levels. Only when this level has been achieved does the PUFA have an effect on the severity and duration of relapses.

The results of this trial are sometimes taken to prove that evening primrose oil does not work. This is not a fair assessment at all. What the trial results do show is that six capsules of evening primrose oil on their own without any additional intake of linoleic acid is not enough to affect plasma levels of linoleate.

Some people have criticized this particular trial on two counts. First, no advice was given about cutting down on saturated fats in the diet. Saturated fats are thought to compete with polyunsaturated fats. Second, the Naudicelle capsules used at that time had orange and black shells, colored by the dye tartrazine. It is known that tartrazine interferes with fatty acid metabolism. Since then, evening primrose oil capsules have been produced in clear gelatin shells.

In everyday life, you are likely to eat a good amount of linoleic acid in addition to taking six capsules of evening primrose oil. This would be in the form of sunflower seed oil margarine, cooking oils such as sunflower or safflower seed oil, and oils rich in linoleic acid for salad dressing. It is a pity that no one has conducted another trial involving evening primrose oil in which these factors are taken into consideration.

Because there has been no scientific evidence in favor of evening primrose oil as a therapy for MS, it is not prescribable and must be bought from health food stores or by mail order from the manufacturers. Many people with MS find evening primrose oil too expensive to buy and don't take it at all.

FISH OILS (SOMETIMES CALLED MARINE OILS)

In the last few years, the spotlight has fallen on the importance of the gamma-linolenic family of essential fatty acids. The richest source of alpha-linolenic acid is oily seafoods.

It is now believed that the best way to take essential fatty acids is as a balance of the linoleic acid family and the alpha-linolenic family in a ratio of approximately 5:1 (5 linoleic acid to 1 alpha-linolenic acid). The wrong balance of the two families of EFAs can create difficulties.

There is nothing very new about research into fish oils. More than thirty years ago, Professor Hugh Sinclair had understood that Eskimos did not get the chronic diseases of western civilization because their intake of fish oils was so high. The type of fat that comes from fish oils is used in the brain and nervous system. That old wives' tale that fish is good for your brain is actually true! It is eicosapentaenoic acid together with arachidonic acid, and not linoleic acid, that is used in the brain.

Many evening primrose oil capsules are now produced in combination with a variety of fish oils. If you buy an evening primrose oil product on its own, it is important to make sure that you are taking enough fish oils or alpha-linolenic acid in another form, e.g., linseeds or split linseeds.

Fish Oil Capsules

Any supplement containing a mixture of fish oils, or cod liver oil.

Vitamin E

It is absolutely vital that you take vitamin E at the same time that you take evening primrose oil. The vitamin E acts as an anti-oxidant. Without anti-oxidants, PUFAs can create harmful peroxides (see "free radicals" on page 78).

Many evening primrose oil capsules contain vitamin E. Some of the cheaper brands do not. So if you buy a brand that is without vitamin E, be sure to take a supplement of vitamin E. (See Chapter 8 on vitamins and minerals.)

FIGURE 9
Alpha-Linolenic Acid Turns into Longer-Chain Fatty Acids, and Then into Series 3 Prostaglandins

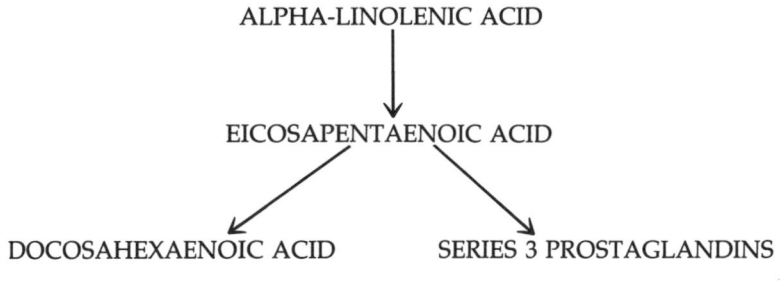

Co-Factors

For evening primrose oil to be metabolized properly, it must be taken with the following vitamins and minerals:

vitamin C
vitamin B_6
vitamin B_3 (better known as nicotinic acid or niacin)
zinc
magnesium

These are described in more detail in the next chapter.

Boosting the Immune System

All of these nutrients, taken together, have the effect of boosting the immune system. This is in contrast to drugs such as steroids, which, although they have short-term success in their anti-inflammatory action, *weaken* the immune system in the long term.

8

Supplements 2: Vitamins, Minerals, Trace Elements, and Amino Acids

There are good reasons to take supplements of vitamins and minerals. First, your diet may not be providing enough. Second, you may need more than a normally healthy person because you have a chronic illness. Third, some specific vitamins and minerals are vital for the biochemical conversion process of essential fatty acids. And last, certain vitamins and minerals are essential if you are taking EFAs to keep them from being oxidated.

Doctors like to tell you that you will be getting enough vitamins and minerals if you are eating a balanced diet. This may not be true for people with MS.

ARMS say that supplements of vitamins and minerals are not necessary if you stick to their EFA diet, which is high in all nutrients including vitamins and minerals. As with all diets, however, many people do *not* stick to them, human frailty being what it is. In their own research, ARMS found that more than a third of people with MS did not comply with the dietary advice given.

In an ideal world, one would eat nutritionally optimal food all the time, and this would be a good source of vitamins and minerals. It is a worthy aim, and I am all in favor of optimal nutrition—I do not believe that supplements should be taken *instead* of eating a healthy diet. A recent survey in the USA found that 60 percent of professional nutritionists, who should know how to eat, regularly took nutritional supplements. My own view is that taking supplements of vitamins and minerals is a sensible insurance policy to be absolutely sure that you are getting enough of them. Doctors specializing in nutritional medicine who have the equipment to do accurate nutritional profiles find that, typically, someone with MS is deficient, sometimes grossly deficient, in vitamin B_6, zinc, and vitamin B_{12}.

Some of the doses in supplements would be much higher than normally found in foods (e.g., vitamin C). The doses recommended in this book for supplements are all higher than the target levels for dietary nutrients set by ARMS.

The following vitamins, minerals, and trace elements are especially important. The reasons for taking each of them will be explained.

Vitamins

Vitamin B_6
Vitamin B_3 (also known as niacin, nicotinamide, or nicotinic
  acid)
Biotin (one of the B vitamins)
All of the B vitamins
Vitamin C
Vitamin E

Minerals and Trace Elements

Zinc
Magnesium
Manganese
Selenium
Vanadium

Phospholipids

Lecithin

The above list is, of course, in addition to evening primrose oil or another form of GLA, plus fish oils, as described in the previous chapter.

THE CO-FACTORS NEEDED FOR EFA SYNTHESIS

A reminder of the metabolic pathway of EFAs (Figure 10) shows just where certain vitamins and minerals are needed to help the process along.

A shortage of any of these co-factors would interfere with the conversion of EFAs. In fact, deficiencies of zinc, magnesium, or vitamin B_6 can actually block the conversion of cis-linoleic acid to gamma-linolenic acid.

There have been some studies to show that, in general, people with MS are low in zinc, magnesium, vanadium, and vitamin B_6. The deficiencies may be a result of MS, rather than being a cause of it.

Dr. Carl Pfeiffer, who runs the Brain Bio Center in Princeton, New Jersey, found that *all* MS patients tested were pyroluric, which simply means that they are losing zinc and vitamin B_6 in the urine. Dr. Pfeiffer found that when he made up the deficiency of zinc and vitamin B_6 and added a supplement of manganese the patients stabilized. (Pfeiffer's dose is 15 mg zinc plus 50 mg vitamin B_6 plus 10 mg manganese, twice a day.)

In the UK, doctors who specialize in nutritional medicine also give their MS patients zinc plus vitamin B_6. Sometimes the dose of zinc can be very high indeed. Injections of vitamin B_{12} are also recommended, weekly or more frequently.

Free Radicals and Anti-Oxidants

Vitamin C, vitamin E, selenium, and the enzyme superoxide dismutase (SOD) are all anti-oxidants. In some circumstances (e.g., high temperatures), the molecules of essential fatty acids accept oxygen atoms more easily. This is part of the oxidation process. The oxidation process chops fatty acids out of the membranes. These oxygen atoms can then detach themselves and fix into another molecule. These unstable molecules that transport oxygen are called free radicals.

Free radicals can be destructive, causing a loss of integrity of the membranes. All functional controls are lost, and anarchy

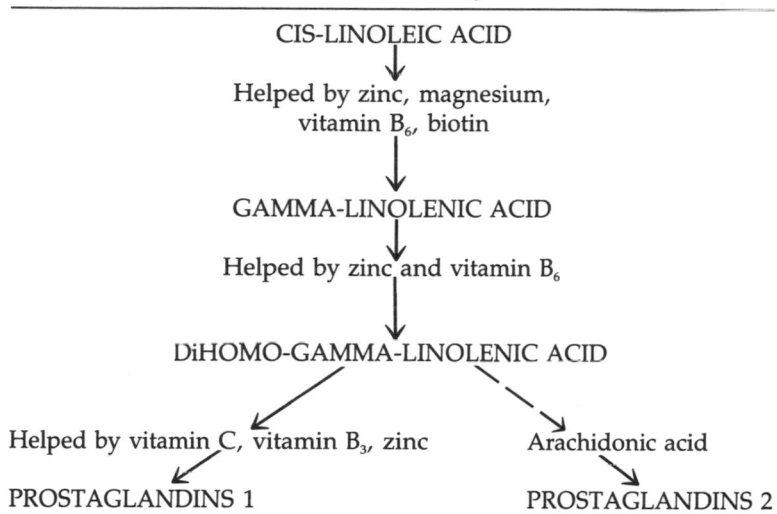

FIGURE 10
The Metabolic Pathway of EFAs

CIS-LINOLEIC ACID

Helped by zinc, magnesium,
vitamin B_6, biotin

GAMMA-LINOLENIC ACID

Helped by zinc and vitamin B_6

DiHOMO-GAMMA-LINOLENIC ACID

Helped by vitamin C, vitamin B_3, zinc   Arachidonic acid

PROSTAGLANDINS 1   PROSTAGLANDINS 2

takes over. Therefore, the whole anti-oxidant system is very important.

The B Group of Vitamins

Vitamin B_6, vitamin B_3 (usually called nicotinic acid), and biotin are essential for the biochemical conversion process of essential fatty acids. The other B vitamins may also be important in MS.

Vitamins B_1 (Thiamine) and B_2 (Riboflavin)

There is some research to show that polyneuritis occurs with vitamin B_1 deficiencies, and people with MS have been found to be low in vitamin B_2. Vitamin B_1 is thought to be effective in improving conditions like neuritis, with numbness of the hands and tingling of the hands and feet. A vitamin B_2 deficiency can be connected with eye problems (e.g., retrobulbar neuritis, blurred vision) and with nervous symptoms like numbness, tremor, and the inability to pass urine. Vitamin B_2 is crucial in the formation of several enzymes. It plays a major role in the metabolism of proteins, fats, and carbohydrates. It enhances the metabolism of vitamin B_6, and there is an interrelationship between vitamins B_2 and B_6.

Vitamin B_3 (Niacin, Nicotinamide, Nicotinic Acid)
It is thought that people with MS are lacking in this vitamin, which forms part of the body's enzyme systems and is essential for the biochemical conversion processes in the body.

Vitamin B_6 (Pyridoxine)
Vitamin B_6 is necessary for the first stages of the biochemical conversion process of essential fatty acids. It also seems to play an important role in the health of muscles and nerves.

Vitamin B_{12}
People with MS need vitamin B_{12} because they are believed to have impaired absorption of this vitamin from the gastrointestinal tract. It therefore has to be given by injection.

Vitamin B_{12} deficiencies can sometimes produce a disease that mimics MS. A shuffling gait or paralysis may occur, but these symptoms are usually associated with severe anemia. As far as MS is concerned, vitamin B_{12} has a role in the maintenance of myelin in the nervous system. It is also needed for folate to be able to work properly.

Pantothenic Acid
In certain laboratory animals, pantothenic acid deficiency has produced loss of the myelin sheath and degenerative changes in the spinal cord and peripheral nerves. The need for pantothenic acid is increased under stress, and it is a good anti-stress supplement.

Choline and Inositol
Choline is involved in the metabolism of fats. It helps in the production of lecithin (phospholipids). Inositol, too, aids in the

metabolism of fats and apparently has some effect on muscular tissue.

Folic Acid

Folic acid is evidently important in helping new cells to form. It is very important in making blood and in keeping the intestines in good condition. It is also vital in maintaining healthy nerve function. A deficiency in folic acid may be the most common vitamin deficiency.

Biotin

Biotin is required by the body to assist in the metabolism of fats. A deficiency of biotin can cause a disturbed nervous system.

Things that Rob You of B Vitamins

The B vitamins are vulnerable to heat, air, and water in cooking. If you cook foods in too much water, the B vitamins will get thrown down the drain with the discarded water. A lot of B_6 and folic acid is destroyed by heat in the cooking process, and some B vitamins get lost when food is exposed to light.

Alcohol, coffee, and other drinks containing caffeine have a nasty way of depleting the body of the B vitamins. These stimulants seem to increase the loss of nearly all nutrients that dissolve in water. Research in the USA has shown that caffeine creates a shortage of inositol in the body.

Many of the B vitamins are also made by bacteria in the intestine, but if you are taking an antibiotic this will destroy the bacteria involved in this process.

The B vitamins are synergistic, which means that they work better when they are taken with each other and with certain other vitamins and minerals (zinc has already been mentioned). Be particularly careful *not* to take vitamin B_1 on its own. All B vitamins must be taken daily as they are not stored in the body.

Dose

The best way to take the B vitamins is in a commercial "B Complex" tablet. In addition, you could take one vitamin B_6 50-mg tablet (not more than twice a day) if the dose of B_6 in the complex tablet is much lower than this. Vitamin B_6 should always be taken with vitamin B complex.

Vitamin C

Vitamin C is not stored in the body, so it has to be taken daily by dietary means. It has two vital functions connected with MS. It stimulates the formation of prostaglandins made from essential fatty acids. The conversion of dihomo-gamma-linolenic acid into prostaglandins 1 is activated by vitamin C, together with zinc and nicotinic acid (B_3). The second vital function of vitamin C is as an anti-oxidant. This is vital when you are eating a diet rich in essential fatty acids. Without taking anti-oxidants as well, essential fatty acids could even be dangerous.

Vitamin C is also well known as a detoxifying agent and as a therapy for infections. It helps the body defend itself against any foreign substance reaching the blood and increases the bacteria-destroying ability of the white blood cells.

The vitamin C content of foods is destroyed by cooking, both by the heat and by the loss in the water thrown away after cooking, so it is a good idea to take supplements of vitamin C as well as including vitamin C–rich foods in your diet to ensure a high daily intake.

Dose: The ARMS target level for vitamin C is 120 mg a day for both men and women. A suitable supplement of vitamin C could contain 1,000 mg or more twice a day. Vitamin C is non-toxic, and there is no risk in taking high doses.

Vitamin E

Vitamin E is essential to prevent oxidation of unsaturated fats to dangerous peroxides. It probably also reduces the conversion of essential fatty acids into toxic substances.

Supplements of evening primrose oil or other products containing GLA *must* be taken with vitamin E. Many of the capsules available already contain vitamin E, but some do not.

Red blood cells break down when essential fatty acids, which form the cell structure, are harmed by oxygen because of a lack of vitamin E. Muscular weakness can occur if the muscles are are not supplied with vitamin E, and the muscles can suffer from an increased content of calcium.

Dose: Supplements of vitamin E could be as high as 600 to 1,000 i.u. per day. The ARMS target is 12 mg a day.

MINERALS AND TRACE ELEMENTS

Zinc

Zinc is an extremely important trace element, as it is part of at least one hundred sixty different enzymes. Indeed, it is the most widely used mineral in the formation of enzymes. These enzymes are involved in digestion, metabolism, and tissue respiration. Zinc is essential for the production of proteins and for the synthesis of DNA—the basis of the genetic code. It also takes a leading role in the processes that ensure normal absorption and function of vitamins, especially the B group.

Zinc is needed in the metabolism of the essential fatty acids from which prostaglandins are produced. This means that the immune system cannot work properly without zinc. Each stage of the metabolic pathway of linoleic acid involves zinc. Zinc has an important role to play in the synthesis of PG1. It is also important in maintaining a balance between prostaglandins 1 and prostaglandins 2.

Zinc plays an important role in the specialization of lymphocytes, the white cells. T lymphocytes mature in the thymus (that's why they are called T lymphocytes). These T lymphocytes are the body's army, so they are essential if the immune system is to defend itself properly. Some of these T lymphocytes become T-killers, which can destroy their targets; others become T-helpers, which can help other white cells make antibodies; and others become T-suppressors, which moderate the manufacture of antibodies. The activity of the thymic hormones is also related to the availablity of zinc.

This vital trace element is mostly found in animal foods. Oysters are the richest source, and meat is a good source. Vegetarians and people who subsist on processed and refined foods may be low in zinc. The cheapest foods tend to be lowest in zinc. There is some evidence that people who have suffered physical injury or disease increase their excretion of zinc. Alcohol, corticosteroids, and the contraceptive pill also cause the loss of zinc from the body.

Zinc and Vitamin B_6

Zinc teams up with vitamin B_6 in the body, particularly for protein synthesis. It seems that our needs for zinc and B_6 are increased in what physiologists call situations of helplessness and hopelessness, which means situations in which one has no control.

Dose: You need to be sure of getting 15 mg of *elemental* zinc twice a day. Read the label of supplements containing zinc carefully, as they can be misleading. (The target level for zinc in the ARMS diet is only 12 mg of zinc a day for both men and women.)

Magnesium

A deficiency of magnesium upsets the nerve-muscle functions and can be associated with tremor, convulsions, over-excitability, and behavioral problems. A group of healthy volunteers who went on a diet deficient in magnesium developed muscle spasms and weakness, involuntary twitching, and inability to control the bladder. These symptoms all went away when they took magnesium again. Some people with MS in the USA reported that supplements of magnesium got rid of foot cramps. Some studies have shown that people with MS are low in magnesium.

Magnesium is needed to help linoleic acid convert to gamma-linolenic acid. A deficiency of magnesium would get in the way of the conversion process at this step.

Magnesium is closely related to calcium and phosphorus in its metabolic functions. Both calcium outside the cells and magnesium inside the cells are important in helping to transmit nerve impulses to muscles.

Dose: 50 mg once a day.

Manganese

Manganese should not be confused with magnesium. The main reason for taking a supplement of manganese is to counterbalance the zinc supplements. As your zinc level goes up, your manganese level goes down. For every 15 mg of zinc you take, you should at the same time take 10 mg of manganese.

In animal studies, a deficiency of manganese has been associated with disturbed balance (ataxia), fatigue, depression, and allergies. In the experience of Dr. Carl Pfeiffer, author of many books about elemental nutrition, all auto-immune diseases respond to manganese.

As a matter of interest, the level of manganese is particularly high in tropical fruits and spices such as clove, cardamom, ginger, turmeric, cinnamon, and black pepper. MS is virtually unknown in countries where these foods are eaten every day.

Dose: 10 mg twice a day.

Selenium

Selenium is a mineral. It is one of the body's protectors, being an anti-oxidant. It is present in an enzyme called glutathione peroxidase (GTP). The various substances that attack cells are rapidly destroyed by GTP before they can cause any damage. Lack of selenium reduces the efficiency of GTP, and body cells are then open to danger. The white blood cells also contain high amounts of GTP. As an anti-oxidant, selenium should be taken together with vitamin C and vitamin E.

People with MS are believed to be low in selenium. The functions of selenium include maintenance of the immune system through the white blood cells; protection against toxic materials such as cadmium and mercury; the production of prostaglandins; an anti-inflammatory effect; protection against free radicals; and a synergistic action with vitamin E in maintaining the functions of mitochondria, the energy-producing apparatus in all body cells.

Dose: 50 µg twice a day. The recommended dietary intake is not to exceed 200 mg a day.

Vanadium

Vanadium is a trace element. People who have MS are thought to be low in vanadium. Deficiency states in animals show up in reduction in red blood cell production, increased blood fat level, and increased blood cholesterol levels. Vanadium has functions in fat metabolism and blood production.

Daily intakes of vanadium in the diet are probably between 100 and 300µg. The best food sources are parsley, radishes, lettuce, strawberries, calf liver, sardines, cucumbers, and apples. There is no need to take vanadium in supplements.

OTHER SUPPLEMENTS*

Lecithin

Lecithin plays a vital role in the metabolism of fats. In her book *Let's Get Well,* Adelle Davis says that autopsy studies on people with MS showed a marked decrease in the lecithin content of the brain and myelin sheath covering the nerves, both of which are normally high in lecithin. The lecithin in people with MS is also, apparently, abnormal, containing saturated instead of un-saturated fats.

Lecithin is continuously produced by the liver, passes into the intestine with bile, and is absorbed into the blood. It aids in the transportation of fats, helps the cells remove fats and cholesterol

---

*There is one spa in Yugoslavia that has earned the reputation of being very beneficial to MS sufferers. Of all the spas in Yugoslavia, it is the only one reputed to have these healing properties for MS. Some scientists have analyzed the spring water and found that it does have special properties and that it contains elements rarely found in spring water. Gornja Trepca has acquired the name of "atomic spa" because it has increased radioactivity. The spring contains such microelements as cesium, rubidium, strontium, and radium and also lithium, cobalt, vanadium, titanium, uranium, radon, manganese, and other constituents. The most unusual element is cesium. It is found here in a concentration very rare in European water. Gornja Trepca is registered with the Yugoslav Ministry of Health as a curative spa center. It is recommended in the treatment of MS by the authorities there.

from the blood, and serves as a structural material for every cell in the body, particularly in the brain and nerves.

Lecithin consists of several substances that require essential fatty acids, choline, and inositol for their structure and numerous other nutrients for their synthesis. If these other raw materials are in short supply, lecithin is not manufactured efficiently in the body. These other nutrients include vitamin B_6 and magnesium.

Dose: Two 200-mg tablets three times a day.

Amino Acids

Until now the emphasis with nutritional supplements has been on vitamins, minerals, and essential fatty acids. One essential metabolite has been missing from this team—amino acids.

Amino acids are the building blocks of proteins. All tissue in the body is made from amino acids—every cell, every muscle, each hair and nail, all of the 15,000 enzymes, and each chemical in the brain is made from amino acids. They are crucial to the biochemistry of the body.

The highly complex molecular logic of our bodies, with its intricate metabolic pathways, needs the right nutrients in the right amounts to function smoothly and efficiently. These nutrients are vitamins, minerals, fatty acids, *and* amino acids and other metabolites derived from them, all working synergistically in harmony.

Amino acids are as important as any of these other nutrients, and a lack of any of them can have a cascade of consequences on health and well-being. The philosophy of doctors specializing in nutritional medicine is that every disorder is the result of metabolic imbalances rather than of a single specific cause. They believe that, just as imbalances can cause disorders, so correcting the metabolic imbalances can put right disorders. Until very recently, amino acids were left out of this equation.

We have already seen what can happen to the body if it is lacking in essential fatty acids, vitamins, and minerals. If the body lacks amino acids, it simply degenerates.

There are twenty-two amino acids capable of producing over

50,000 different protein structures. Eight of these are called essential amino acids because the body cannot make them. To obtain essential amino acids, you must eat the protein foods. These eight are called phenylalanine, tryptophan, methionine, lysine, leucine, isoleucine, valine, and threonine.

With these eight amino acids, the body can use metabolic pathways to synthesize all of the others. The nonessential amino acids include tyrosine, asparagine, ornithine, histidine, glutamic acid, glutamine, proline, and glycine.

Without animo acids, human life would not exist. They supply the raw materials for maintaining the genetic code—DNA—as well as for repairing damaged tissue, for cell division, for making enzymes, for building new connective tissue, and for making hormones, which regulate bodily processes and neurotransmitters. It makes sense to take amino acids for multiple sclerosis, a degenerative disease in which you need all the help you can get to repair damaged tissue.

Amino acids are not drugs and are not toxic. They are like the broken-down molecules of food. They cannot do you any harm, and they might well do you some good. People with MS who have taken "free-form" amino acids report an immediate boost in energy and an end to that draining symptom of MS, fatigue.

Why You Should Take Amino Acid Supplements

If you are eating a good healthy diet with lots of protein, such as meat, fish, and eggs, you may wonder why you should be taking amino acid supplements at all. The answer is that your body may not be processing protein properly. Faulty protein digestion can result in partial amino acid deficiency, even if you are eating a lot of protein in your daily diet. If you are suffering from fatigue and if your body is showing some signs of degeneration, then the protein you are eating may not be reaching the places where it is most needed.

One possible cause of this is not chewing your food properly. Other possible causes are factors that can decrease the output of digestive chemicals, such as emotional stress, junk food, not enough exercise, viruses, pollution, injury, drugs (e.g., cannabis), and genetic disorders.

Children are usually told to chew their food properly, and there are sound reasons for this. Chewing properly tears the food apart, breaks it down, and helps to release digestive substances. The more thoroughly you chew, the more nutrients your body will absorb. If you gobble your food and bolt it down, the acids and enzymes don't have as large a surface area to work on. When the food reaches the gut, less of it is digested. As a result, fewer amino acids are absorbed into the body to carry out vital protein synthesis.

Once this happens, you are caught in a vicious circle because one of the important roles of protein synthesis is to manufacture digestive enzymes. If there is poor protein synthesis, there will be fewer enzymes to digest the food, and fewer amino acids will be released from the food to build the body's tissues.

The domino effect from this can be quite dramatic, as amino acids have such varied and vital functions. As the number of amino acids drops, there is an effect on hormone production, with less insulin to regulate blood sugar levels, less epinephrine to help you cope with stress, less thyroxine to carry out body metabolism, and less thymosin to stimulate the immune system. Body tissues show the signs of a shortage of amino acids—muscle tone will fade, skin will slacken, nails will become soft and split.

A shortage of amino acids can greatly affect your mood and well-being. You are likely to get tired easily and to suffer from bouts of anxiety and depression. You are more susceptible to disease, and you may show signs of premature aging.

How to Take Amino Acids
The best way to take amino acids is to take supplements of free-form amino acids in either powder form or capsules. Free-form amino acids are amino acids that require no digestion whatsoever. They are absorbed straight through the intestinal walls and into the bloodstream. Free-form amino acid treatment is very fast; some people report feeling the effects virtually imme-

diately. The most likely effects with MS are a boost in energy levels, a lessening of fatigue, and the disappearance of hypoglycemia.

Free-form amino acids can help particularly against allergies and autoimmune diseases, of which multiple sclerosis can be counted as one. They work by strengthening the natural metabolic reactions of the body, with the help of vitamin and mineral co-factors (especially vitamins B_3, B_6, and C).

Some doctors who have been using free-form amino acids in the treatment of multiple sclerosis include all of the sulfur-based amino acids because these work by improving the state of body tissue. These amino acids are methionine, taurine, cysteine, and cystine. Methionine also works to rid the body of mercury and other heavy metals (lead, cadmium) because it is a chelator, latching on to the toxic metals and escorting them out of the body.

To treat yourself, you can buy free-form amino acids in a health food shop or by mail order. If possible, however, it is better to consult a nutritionally oriented doctor. The doctor will be able to give you some specific tests to determine your amino acid profile to formulate a prescription that is tailor-made to your specific needs. There is a particular test known as the urinary amino test that can analyze the amino acids in your urine and identify any deficits.

Ideally, free-form amino acids should be taken on an empty stomach twice a day, first thing in the morning and last thing at night, or as directed by your physician. If you are taking the powdered form, dissolve half a teaspoon in half a tumbler of water, washed down with another half tumbler of water. Always take amino acids with the vitamin and mineral co-factors, as described earlier in this chapter.

As well as boosting your energy levels, free-form amino acids should have the effect of reducing the sensation of feeling weak with hunger, the hypoglycemia common in MS caused by low blood sugar levels. The hormone insulin regulates blood sugar levels, and insulin production is dependent upon amino acids.

Urinary Amino Tests and Suppliers of Free-Form Amino Acids

USA

Medabolics
22318 NE 169th Street
Brush Prairie, WA
 98606
(206)254-2202
[Outside Washington
 (800)257-1121]

Doctor's Data
30 West 101
Roosevelt Road
West Chicago, IL 60195

Smith Klyne
Bio-Science Laboratories
7600 Tyrone Avenue
Van Nuys, CA 91405

Bionostics Inc.
4736 Main Street, Suite
 10A
P.O. Drawer 400
Lisle, IL 60532
(312)960-4045

AUSTRALIA

Munashi Aminos
361 Beaconsfield Parade
St. Kilda
Melbourne, Victoria
 3182
(3)534-5251

Xandria Williams
366 Military Road
Cremorne, NSW 2090
(2)290-4771

Recommended Reading
Erdmann, R., and Jones, M. *The Amino Revolution*. Century Paperbacks.

Co-enzyme Q10

Another new nutrient on the market that might be of benefit to someone with multiple sclerosis is called co-enzyme Q10. Like germanium, it gives a boost to the immune system.

Co-enzyme Q10 (co-Q10) plays a vital role in the utilization of oxygen by body cells and is therefore essential for the health of all human tissues and organs. Co-Q10 also improves exercise tolerance by helping muscle cells use oxygen.

Although it is found in certain foods, including beef, sardines, spinach, and peanuts, co-Q10 is difficult to extract from these sources. Co-Q10 is synthesized in the body, but this ability seems to decline with age and when the immune system is not working well, so deficiencies of this nutrient can occur in people who have MS. Apparently approximately 12 million people in Japan take co-Q10, and it is gaining ground as a nutrient that will help retard the ageing process.

Although most of the tests have thus far been done on animals, co-Q10 has been proven safe to take. However, one has to be cautious about the claims made. If you decide to try it, the best dosage is probably 30 mg a day.

Lactobacillus acidophilus (or Similar Products)

The intestines are populated with two predominant groups of bacteria, the putrefactive Bacteroides and the beneficial Bifidobacteria. The aim of taking supplements such as *Lactobacillus acidophilus*, probion, or similar products is to promote the correct balance between the two main types of bacteria.

Degenerative conditions like multiple sclerosis are believed by some practitioners to be connected with an imbalance of the putrefactive Bacteroides against the healthier Bifidobacteria, with a consequent build-up of toxicity in the system. A disease such as MS indicates that the inner environment of the body is unbalanced, with a depletion of oxygen and essential nutrients and autointoxication. Taking supplements of acidophilus will help reestablish healthy intestinal flora.

One of the big advantages of taking acidophilus or a similar product is that it will help bring about regular and easy bowel movements (see section on constipation, page 207). Taking acidophilus will also help bring *Candida albicans* under control.

Dose: One 500-mg acidophilus capsule one to three times a day. (If taking a similar product, follow the directions on the container.)

CONCLUSION

Here is a complete list of supplements beneficial to people with MS, together with their suggested doses.

- Evening primrose oil capsules—Ideally, nine capsules a day. Three capsules of 500 mg, three times a day with meals.
- Fish oil capsules—1,000 mg of fish lipid, one capsule a day. Or combine evening primrose oil with fish oil in one capsule.
- Vitamin C—Up to 1 gram per tablet. One tablet three times a day.
- Vitamin E—Up to 1000 i.u. per tablet. One tablet three times a day.
- B Complex (all of the B vitamins in balance)—Any commercial product should supply adequate amounts in the right ratios. One tablet three times a day.
- Vitamin B_6—50 mg once or twice a day (no more).
- Vitamin B_{12}—Injections once a week or more often of 1 mg of hydroxycobalamin.
- Zinc—15 mg at least of elemental zinc twice a day.
- Magnesium—50 mg a day.
- Manganese—10 mg twice a day.
- Selenium—50 µg twice a day.
- Lecithin—Two tablets of 200 mg, three times a day.
- Free-form amino acids—½ teaspoon in water twice a day.
- Organic germanium—50 mg a day.
- Co-enzyme Q10—30 mg a day.
- Acidophilus (or similar product)—Up to three doses of 500 mg a day.

It is possible to find vitamin and mineral products that combine some of these nutrients in one tablet, which saves the bother of having to take several different supplements. All of these fatty acids, vitamins, minerals, trace elements, and amino acids work together as a team, so it is important to take them in the right balance and not to take huge amounts of certain nutrients and nothing of other ones.

The listed doses are approximations. If you can see a nutritionally qualified practitioner who can give you an accurate nutritional profile, then supplements and doses can be tailor-made to your particular needs.

9

Food Allergies and Clinical Ecology

In recent years, the whole subject of food allergies has gained in popularity and even in an acceptance by some doctors. This whole area is sometimes called clinical ecology.

CLINICAL ECOLOGY

This is an American term that originated in Chicago, thanks to the pioneering work of Dr. Theron Randolph. Clinical ecology is the study of how the environment promotes disease or ill health in individuals. The most common environmental factors that can bring about ill health are foods and chemicals. The aim of a clinical ecologist is to use various techniques to pinpoint the foods, chemicals, or other substances that might be causing the problem, to exclude those toxic substances from the patient's lifestyle, and to detoxify the body. This must be done on an individual basis, as one substance can be perfectly benign to one person yet toxic to another.

THE DEFINITION OF "ALLERGY"

There may be many doctors who take issue with the word "allergy" being used in the way I am using it in this book. Most immunologists take the view that "allergy" involves only those reactions in which a specific immunological (antigen-antibody) reaction can be demonstrated. This is the narrow definition of the word "allergy."

A wider definition of allergy includes supersensitivity to substances that has no known immunological basis. This more generalized term is in keeping with the word "allergy" originally coined by the Austrian physician Clement von Pirquet at the beginning of this century. Von Pirquet himself stated that the term "allergy" involved the general concept of changed reactivity.

This wider definition of allergy, which does not necessarily involve antigen-antibody reactions, is in current usage today. It is in this broad sense that the term "allergy" is used in this book.

FOOD ALLERGIES

Testing for food allergies is one part of the job of a clinical ecologist. Another part is to test for other things that could be toxic to the individual, such as mercury in your dental fillings, cigarette smoke, or chemicals (pesticides, for example).

Over the last fifteen years or so there have been some very well documented individual successes of people with MS who have excluded certain foods from their diet, and their MS has improved—sometimes dramatically—as a result. Everything in this chapter is based on "anecdotal evidence"—a number of individual case histories added together. We are now in the field of "alternative medicine," where practitioners take issue with the conventional scientific method and the approach of suppressing symptoms. As each person with MS may be allergic to a different set of foods and substances, it would be impossible to set up an orthodox controlled trial. However, many of the practitioners of clinical ecology are doctors trained in orthodox medicine who have gone over to the other camp because they have become disillusioned with various aspects of orthodox medicine.

The Multiple Sclerosis Society, both in the UK and the USA, dismisses the field of clinical ecology as being unproven and unscientific. It is a pity that both groups take this attitude. I have met several people who swear by the food allergy approach and whose lives have improved immeasurably as a result of excluding the foods and substances to which they were sensitive. If you want hard proof, you won't find it here, but it is wise to be open-minded on this topic as hard proof is never likely to be forthcoming in this realm.

Dr. Patrick Kingsley, one of the leading doctors practicing clinical ecology in the UK, has treated hundreds of MS patients. At a conservative estimate, he claims that more than 50 percent of these MS patients have improved as a result of excluding the foods and substances to which they were found to be reacting. In other words, they have gotten better, rather than getting worse. As well as excluding allergic foods, doctors practicing clinical ecology prescribe a wide range of nutritional supplements for their MS patients (see previous chapter).

Test Yourself for Food Allergies before Starting Any Diet for MS

If the food allergists are right, you should test yourself for your particular food allergies *before* starting on the ARMS essential fatty acid diet, the Swank low fat diet, or any other diet suggested for MS. If you are allergic to milk, for example, you should not eat *any* milk products, no matter how skimmed or low fat they may be. You might find you are allergic to perfectly healthy foods that are recommended on the ARMS diet, such as tomatoes, green peppers, apples, or bananas.

Food Allergies and MS

When your body's immune system has gone wrong, as with MS, you can show abnormal reactions to foods that a normally healthy person could eat without any bad effects. Allergy symptoms include tiredness after meals, palpitations, headache, nausea, bloating, a high pulse rate, and sweating. In MS, the symptoms can also include cold legs, constricted breathing, difficulties with vision, lethargy, depression, and a rapid onset of MS symptoms.

Are Food Allergies the Cause of MS or the Result of Having MS?
It is not clear whether food and other allergies are the *result* of having MS or in some way are involved in *causing* the disease.

For a long time, naturopaths have believed that toxic substances cause chronic illness. At long last, some conventionally trained doctors are catching up with the naturopaths and looking scientifically at how food and other substances can be toxic to an individual.

The offending food may give you a specific symptom. It could be, for example, that cane sugar makes your eyes go hazy or that grapefruit juice makes your speech more slurred.

Thanks to the work of Dr. Richard Mackarness, who wrote *Not All in the Mind* (Pan), we know that the foods you crave most and eat most habitually are likely to be the very foods to which you are allergic. This is unfortunate but true. In his book *Chemical Victims*, Dr. Mackarness also made people aware of "masked allergies." Roughly, this means that you are addicted to various foods and substances, and you get symptoms when you don't have them—rather like symptoms of withdrawal from a drug.

Orthodox doctors tend to dismiss the possibility of food allergies, saying that, once eaten, all foods get broken down in the digestive process to the same basic molecules anyway, so it shouldn't make any difference what you eat. These doctors also tend to take umbrage at the misuse of the word "allergy." Doctors who specialize in nutritional medicine or clinical ecology, however, are convinced that there is a link between eating food to which you may be sensitive and a whole range of different symptoms.

Some neurologists have also had to join the food allergy camp when they have seen the evidence with their own eyes. One such is the American neurologist Dr. Robert Soll, who now runs a clinic in Iowa where he treats MS patients using allergy techniques.

Dr. Soll evolved the idea that "individuals with Multiple Sclerosis frequently display a profile of numerous allergies. . . . This condition might . . . cause the absorption of endotoxin from the intestines and an attack of MS." Dr. Soll's definition of endotoxins is bacterial poisons produced by an infection. In his book *MS: Something Can Be Done and You Can Do It* (Contemporary Books), he says:

The intestinal tract may represent a large reservoir of endotoxin, and very small quantities of the substance may be absorbed through a weakened, inflamed intestinal wall as would result from the ingestion of allergic foods. Thus, an infection, which would cause a greater release of endotoxin into the bloodstream, not only causes fever and cold hands and cold feet, but also an acute exacerbation of MS. On the other hand, inflammation of the bowel wall resulting in absorption of endotoxin could produce a slow, cumulative adverse effect day after day, contributing to the slow, downhill course we see so often in MS patients.

In his book, Dr. Soll cites several cases of people with MS who have very dramatic "before and after" stories. In each case, he isolated the foods to which these people were allergic and the foods were banned. These patients were also treated with antibiotics each time they had an infection.

Possible Mechanisms for Certain Foods Causing Allergies

The mechanism for certain foods causing allergies in some people with MS probably involves the gut. Semi-digested food is getting through permeable intestine walls. Perhaps this permeability is caused by a proliferation of candida (see page 107).

Damage to the Intestinal Mucosa
The intestinal mucosa may be damaged because of a cow's milk allergy that began very early in the person's life, perhaps even as early as the first days. In western societies, the period around birth is disturbed dramatically. Ideally, the baby should be able to suck at its mother's breast within the first hour or so after the birth. The baby's first food is colostrum. Colostrum contains special antibodies (IgA) able to protect the intestinal mucosa.

However, few babies get the optimal amount of colostrum in their first days of life. Many babies born in a hospital—even those whose mothers want to breastfeed—are given a small bottle of formula. In effect, they are given foreign proteins, to which they may become sensitive for the rest of their lives.

Malabsorption
If there is damage to the lining of the gastrointestinal tract and food is seeping through the gut walls, the food you eat is not being absorbed properly. If malabsorption is a problem, then the body will be deficient in minerals, vitamins, and trace elements. This in itself would have a fairly catastrophic cascade of consequences. Too much tea or coffee can also block the absorption of all of the minerals and some vitamins.

Abnormal Immune Reactions
The immune system also seems to be involved in the mechanism of food allergies. In a complex way that is not fully understood, the immune system decides that these food substances are foreign bodies and sets the troops in motion against body tissues. It is thought that the immunoglobulins are involved in this. These are large protein molecules manufactured by special white cells, the B lymphocytes.

Immunoglobulins are proteins, and their detailed chemical structure is designed to bind specifically to the chemicals or bacteria defined as foreign, i.e., nonself. Under normal circumstances, the body is able to recognize itself and so does not make immunoglobulins (or antibodies) that destroy its own structures.

Recent research shows that there is an abnormality of immunoglobulins in 54.5 percent of MS patients. No one has yet forged any link between the fact and the possibility of food allergies.

Proliferation of Candida *and Leaky Mucous Membranes*
There is evidence that there is a connection between yeast and MS. No one is saying that *Candida* is the cause of MS, merely that there is a connection and that, once candidiasis is treated, the patient's condition will improve.

Candida albicans is a yeast-like organism, known to laymen as thrush. *C. albicans* figures prominently in the intestinal tract of humans. Under normal circumstances, *C. albicans* is an innocent bystander, but trouble starts when the *Candida* changes from its normal yeast-like form to a mycelian fungal form. The yeast-like state is nothing to worry about, but the fungal form produces long, root-like mycelia that can penetrate the mucous membrane of the intestine. This penetration can lead to leaky mucous membranes in the digestive tract. This leakage allows incompletely digested substances (e.g., proteins from the diet) to come into direct contact with the immune system. This is why people with a chronic overgrowth of *Candida albicans* often have many food and other allergies.

As well as causing a leaky intestinal mucous membrane, *Candida* also produces a specific toxin called *Candida* toxin. This can weaken the entire immune system and make it less able to deal with allergy problems. (See page 107 for more on candida.)

The Foods to Which People with MS Are Most Commonly Allergic

The foods to which people with MS are most often allergic are

- milk and all dairy products
- yeast (in bread, etc.)
- all fungi (mushrooms, etc.) and fermented products (e.g., vinegar)
- sugar
- potatoes
- tea and anything with tannin

Dr. Patrick Kingsley, who has had more experience in this field than any other doctor in the UK, finds that wheat, barley, oats, and rye (the gluten grains, see page 118) are not commonly foods to which people with MS are allergic. However, some of the foods made with these grains do contain *yeast*, and this could be the problem. Dr. Kingsley also finds that chemicals do not feature very prominently with MS patients, although mercury in dental fillings is a common allergen (see next chapter). Other doctors, however, in both the USA and the UK, would also include

- wheat
- red meat

- fruits
- some vegetables and
- caffeine

in the top ten list of foods to which people with MS are most commonly allergic.

Remember that different foods affect different people differently. Even so, be very suspicious of milk, all dairy products, all sugars, yeast and all fungi (e.g., mushrooms), fruit, wheat, red meat, tea, and vegetables.

If you change your attitude to the culprit foods and think of them as poisons, it's not so hard to give them up completely. If you identify chemical pollutants, the same thing applies. Change your lifestyle to avoid them completely.

What to Avoid on a Cow's Milk–free Diet

Cow's milk (even in very small quantities)
Creamed foods
Creamed sauces
Fresh cream
Cow's milk cheeses of every description
Cow's milk yogurt
Custard
Milk chocolate and some dark chocolate
Butter
Dairy ice cream
Condensed milk
Dried evaporated milk
Powdered milk
Malted milk
Ovaltine
Drinking chocolate
Manufactured salad dressings
Batter
Soups with added milk
Most margarines, because they contain whey (only a very few
   do not)

Foods fried in butter
Cakes, biscuits, and bread with milk in them
Any packaged foods containing milk powder, lactose, whey, or
   casein

If your symptoms improve on a cow's milk–free diet, you can
introduce either goat's milk or its products (e.g., cheese and
yogurt) OR soya milk, but not both at the same time. Ewe's milk
can also be tried.

Remember—read labels!

What to Avoid on a Yeast-free and Sugar-free Diet

Foods that contain yeast as an additive ingredient: biscuits,
   breads, pastries, cakes and cake mixes, flour enriched with
   vitamins from yeast, and meat fried in crumbs
The following contain yeast or yeast-like substances because of
   their nature or the nature of their manufacture and prepara-
   tion: mushrooms, cheeses, and vinegars such as apple, pear,
   cider, grape, and malt vinegars (although some vinegar is pure
   chemical acetic acid, which could be allowed if you could find
   some and be sure about it). These vinegars should be avoided
   in their original state as well as in such foods as mayonnaise,
   olives, pickles, sauerkraut, horseradish, french dressing, and
   tomato sauce. Also avoid bouillon cubes, yeast extracts, and
   gravy mixes.
Fermented drinks: whiskey, gin, wine, brandy, rum, vodka,
   beer; in fact, *all* alcoholic drinks
Malted products: cereals, most chocolates, and malted milk
   drinks
Citrus fruit juices, either frozen or canned, melons; only home-
   squeezed fruit juices are yeast-free.
Many vitamin products are derived from yeast.
Because yeasts feed on sugar and carbohydrate, sugar in all
   forms *must* be avoided: white and brown sugar, honey, maple
   syrup, golden syrup, sweets, toffees, chocolates, candies, ice

cream, cookies, puddings, drinks with added sugar such as sodas, orange drinks, lemonade, Coca-Cola, Pepsi Cola, and virtually all carbonated drinks, including bitter lemon and tonic water. As so many people crave sugar, when you start on a sugar-free diet avoid all sugar substitutes such as saccharin, NutraSweet, and so on, or you will never lose your sweet tooth.

White flour in all forms (such as bread, biscuits, puddings, pasta, cakes), which is so heavily refined that yeasts treat it like sugar.

What to Avoid on a Tannin-free Diet

Tea, Indian and China
Dark-skinned grapes and plums and their dried fruits, e.g., currants, raisins, and prunes
All drinks made from the above fruits, e.g., dark sherry, brandy, red wine, and nonalcoholic drinks from the dark grape

You may have sultanas, herbal teas that are tannin-free (check the labels), and fruit juices that are yeast-free and sugar-free.

What to Avoid on a Totally Caffeine-free Diet

Coffee of all sorts, pure ground, bagged, percolated, and instant; nearly all decaffeinated coffees contain a little caffeine, so avoid them as well
Chocolate, cocoa, chocolate drinks
Coca-Cola and all cola drinks
Mocha frosting on cakes
Some painkillers contain caffeine, so check labels.

It is probably not wise to drink chicory instead, so avoid coffee substitutes that contain chicory.

MS, Sinusitis, and Milk Allergy

In early 1986, there was a flurry of interest about the connection between MS and sinusitis. A paper and correspondence on the subject were published in the *Lancet*, a British medical journal. Professor George Dick and Dr. Derek Gray had found that, of one hundred thirty-five patients with MS in sixteen physicians' practices, 65.9 percent had histories of sinusitis. They found that nasopharyngeal infections and chronic sinusitis were seventeen times more common in the MS patients than in the controls. These figures strongly suggest that there is an association between sinusitis and MS. The doctors conducting this study observed that the peak of sinusitis occurred one year before the first attack of MS.

Professor Dick and Dr. Gray believe that sinusitis and MS may be causally associated because sinusitis and sinomucosal damage precede MS. They also note that sinusitis is common in children aged five to ten. Whatever is it that causes MS is supposed to happen during the first fifteen years of life.

A naturopath or a clinical ecologist faced with a patient with sinusitis would immediately suspect a milk allergy. According to Dr. Patrick Kingsley, "Sinusitis is a clear indication of a milk allergy."

It is very sad that conventionally trained doctors regard suggestions such as this as rubbish. I think that it is foolish to dismiss out of hand such startling correlations—that most people with MS suffer from milk allergy and that 65 percent of people with MS have chronic recurrent sinusitis.

Surely it would be sensible to test anyone with MS who gets chronic sinusitis for milk allergy as the next step in the investigations? Removing milk and milk products from the diet of these patients might have benefits both for their sinusitis and also for their MS.

Early weaning is another factor that can explain the frequency of cow's milk allergy in our society. Babies are fed cow's milk before their digestive systems are ready for anything except mother's milk. This early allergy to cow's milk has long-term consequences and paves the way for allergies later in life. Of all the foods to which MS people are allergic, cow's milk is at the top of the list.

Sugar and MS

Another food in the "Top Ten" list to which people with MS are allergic is sugar. If someone takes 100 grams of sugar in the form of glucose, fructose, sucrose, honey, or even orange juice, there is a significant drop in the efficiency of white blood cells defending the body. The body's defense system reaches the nadir of weakness two hours after someone eats any of these foods.

These particular white blood cells, called neutrophil phagocytes, form about 60 to 70 percent of the total white blood cells. The effect of sugar leaves the body open to invaders. The more sugar given, the more the immune system is inhibited. It is thought that the effect is the result of increased insulin activity, which competes with vitamin C for transport binding sites in the body.

Hypoglycemia

A symptom not usually associated with multiple sclerosis is hypoglycemia—low blood sugar. The person may feel light-headed and weak and may crave something sweet.

The worst thing you can do to alleviate hypoglycemia is to eat something sweet, such as a candy bar or cookies. This simply sets you up to endlessly repeat the pattern. If you do eat a candy bar, your blood sugar will shoot up temporarily, but it will quickly drop down to a low level again, leaving you hypoglycemic, weak, and craving something sweet.

Fluctuating blood sugar levels are a sure sign that there is something wrong nutritionally that needs to be sorted out, with a correct diet plus vitamin and mineral supplements. Instead of going for sugar-laden foods, eat complex carbohydrates, like potatoes in their jackets, which will give a much slower release-type of sugar and help keep your blood sugar levels more stable. Once you stop eating sugar altogether, cut out all junk foods, switch to a healthy, nutritious diet, and take supplements, hypoglycemia as a symptom should disappear completely.

CANDIDA AND MS

Intestinal candidiasis is a major cause of food allergy. Once this is treated, patients complaining of food allergies often improve.

The link between *Candida* and MS was discussed by an American, William G. Crook, M.D., in his book *The Yeast Connection* (published by Professional Books). It was another American, Dr. Orion Truss, who was the first ecologist to recognize the problem of candidiasis.

In *The Yeast Connection*, Dr. Crook mentions several cases of patients with MS who, from their medical history, seemed good candidates for anti-*Candida* treatment. In all of the cases described in his book, the MS symptoms improved as the candidiasis was treated.

The following case history comes from the book *Nutritional Medicine* by Dr. Stephen Davies and Dr. Alan Stewart (Pan Books Ltd., 1987). It illustrates how successful a nutritional approach to multiple sclerosis can be.

> Susan was a 29-year-old mother of two who had developed blurred vision, pins and needles, loss of balance, and weakness in the legs and one hand. She had been diagnosed as having Multiple Sclerosis. Full history-taking revealed that she almost certainly had chronic yeast (candida) problems. Nutritional assessment showed multiple nutrient deficiencies, despite a sensible "well-balanced" diet, suggesting a problem with absorption of nutrients. She also had tell-tale signs of food allergy (gut symptoms, eczema in childhood, migraine). Treating her for chronic candidiasis, treating her for food allergies, and correcting her nutritional deficiencies, including vitamin B_{12} injections (as she was found to be functionally deficient in it) resulted in a marked improvement, to the point that she became symptom-free within a month of commencing treatment. Whilst spontaneous remissions are quite common in Multiple Sclerosis, this case is probably a demonstration of how, after removing certain "loads" (deficiencies, candida, food allergy), the body is better able to heal itself. One and a half years later Susan

is still symptom-free, with no evidence of any recurrence according to her six-monthly check-ups with a neurologist. Furthermore, she feels fitter than at any time during her adult life.

What Can Make Someone Sensitive to *Candida*?

Antibiotics

The story can usually be traced to the patient's childhood, when there may have been recurrent infections—such as urinary tract infections or sinusitis—which had been treated with antibiotics. Antibiotics are very nonselective about which bacteria they kill— they destroy all of them, both good and bad. This upsets the delicate balance of bacteria.

The Contraceptive Pill

The artificial hormones in contraceptive pills disturb many processes in the body. The known metabolic abnormalities produced by the pill include zinc deficiency, too much copper, altered liver function, changes in many hormonal levels, and gross changes in the function of many enzymes. Many women with MS who have candidiasis also take the pill.

The pill alters and depresses the immune system and changes the acidity of vaginal secretions. This often results in thrush.

Sulfonamide Drugs

These drugs are described for conditions such as cystitis (a urinary tract infection). Again, patients who have MS and who have *Candida* sensitivity are frequently found to have taken sulfonamide drugs.

Steroid Drugs

Candidiasis is more likely in patients who have been receiving large doses of steroids. It is quite common for patients to be given oral steroids when they have an attack of MS. The contraceptive pill is also a steroid drug.

It is not uncommon for someone with MS, especially women,

to have been treated with antibiotics and sulfonamide drugs and have been on the contraceptive pill in the years before the diagnosis of MS.

Immunosuppressive Drugs
People who already have something wrong with their immune systems are more open to candidiasis. The irony is that they are doubly at risk if they are also taking immunosuppressive drugs.

At a recent symposium on candidiasis, an American physician, Dr. Jack Remington, said: "When we use corticosteroids, antibiotics, and cytotoxic drugs in such quantities, we are adding insult to injury. We have to use these drugs, of course, but they cause as much immunosuppression as the underlying disease."

The Signs and Symptoms of Chronic Candidiasis

The most common sign of *Candida* is thrush. Thrush is an acute infection or overgrowth of *Candida*. In children, it can occur in the mouth and gastrointestinal tract. In men, it can show up as a sore penis. In women, it is a sore vagina, with a white discharge. Thrush can result from a course of antibiotics.

With chronic candidiasis, the symptoms are almost endless. They range from vaginal irritation, to malaise, to headache.

Once the body has chronic candidiasis, it is unbalanced and predisposed to a variety of ecological problems, including food allergies and other sensitivities.

Treatment

You can find out whether you are sensitive to *Candida* by the same techniques as are used to detect food allergies. *Candida*, like all forms of yeast, loves sugar and moist places. The most common treatment is to exclude from your diet all yeast, all sugars, white flour, cakes, cookies, coffee, alcohol, tea, mushrooms, and cheese. Also, do not eat anything moldy.

An anti-fungal drug called Nystatin* is sometimes prescribed. Doctors who specialize in nutritional medicine would probably also recommend vitamin and mineral supplements, plus evening primrose oil.

Acidophilus is sometimes prescribed to restore the bacteria in the gut to the right balance. Acidophilus is a friendly bacteria found in such foods as live yogurt. However, if you were allergic to milk products you could not take live yogurt. Acidophilus is available in tablet or powder form.

TESTING YOURSELF FOR FOOD ALLERGIES

If you think that you may be allergic to any foods or chemicals, the first thing to do is to get yourself tested for this. In the last few years, tests for food allergies have progressed by leaps and bounds. Until very recently, the only way to find out to which foods you were allergic was to go through the laborious process of going on a cleansing fast and then trying each food one by one. This is still an effective self-help method and cheaper than the other alternatives, but it does take quite a long time and is better done under supervision.

The Do-It-Yourself Approach

The principle behind testing for food allergies is that you can find out to which foods you are allergic only if you go on a strict cleansing fast first to clear impurities from the body. Some doctors recommend a complete fast, but others think that it is safe to start with a cleansing diet of low risk foods.

The Cleansing Diet—Eating Only Low Risk Foods
For five to seven days, go on a cleansing fast eating only low risk foods. The low risk foods, to which very few people are allergic, are lamb, pears, cod, trout, flounder, carrots, zucchini, avocados, string beans, parsnips, rutabagas, and turnips. For

---

*Dr. Stephen Davies, co-author of *Nutritional Medicine*, has a note of caution about Nystatin. He says: "In some situations, anti-candida treatment with Nystatin can cause an acute exacerbation of the condition, so one should progress very cautiously in MS."

these five to seven days, these foods can be eaten in any quantity.

While you are casting off toxins into the bloodstream, you will probably not feel very well. That will have passed by the fifth day. On the sixth day, you should feel well enough to start testing the foods.

Testing the Foods, One by One
At the end of the five to seven days, you can begin testing other foods, one by one. This is not as arduous as it sounds. Once you have passed a food as safe, you can continue to eat it, together with your new food. So you could be eating large and varied meals within a matter of days. There is no limit on quantity.

Begin with foods that many people find safe, i.e., they do not react to them. This list includes broccoli, beef, rice, melon, pineapple, lettuce, apples, grapes, and chicken.

Introduce these one per meal. Separate the meals by five to six hours. Watch for a reaction, which can normally be expected to happen during this period of time. Allow two days to test wheat, corn, oats, and rye, as they can have a delayed reaction.

Foods from the same food family should be spaced out. They should not be introduced within four days of each other.

By testing new foods one at a time, you can easily see if a food gives you any symptoms. If you get no reaction, you can add that food to the next meal. For example, if you had tested lamb safely and rice safely, you could eat lamb, rice, and leeks on the next day for lunch. You would only be testing the leeks at that time, but if you got any reaction, you would know it must be the leeks.

If you do get a reaction, you should not test a new food until you feel well again to avoid confusing the whole test. You might have to wait as long as three days. If you do get a certain reaction, it is wise to retest that food but not for at least another five days or more.

If you break the diet once, you might have to start all over again. You should stick to each day's foods rigidly and eat nothing else—no sauces, flavorings, etc.

This food allergy test contains many foods with saturated fat. You may feel that it is worthwhile to include them in the test to see what kind of reaction you have. Cut the fat off the lamb during the first five days. If you are taking dietary supplements, watch out for additives such as sugar or yeast. Gelatin-covered capsules can be taken throughout the test.

Isolating the Allergen
The important thing about testing foods one by one is that it isolates individual ingredients. You may, for example, feel ill after eating a piece of cake—but what in the cake is making you feel bad? It could be the cane sugar, or the white flour, or the butter, or indeed the cherries on the top.

With bread, you could find that you are allergic to the yeast, rather than the wheat. Be particularly careful about sugar. Beet sugar and cane sugar are not the same thing, and you could react differently to each.

Do not think that foods must be safe because they are "natural." It is possible for tomatoes, potatoes, bananas, almonds, or peanuts, for example, to give you an allergic reaction, even though they are not refined or processed or in any way adulterated.

Needless to say, the process of testing for food allergies is almost impossible socially. If you go anywhere, it is safest to take a picnic of "safe" foods with you, and explain the reason to your hostess. It is too risky eating out as you do not know what the well-meaning cook might have added in the way of sauces.

You must also avoid all alcoholic drinks. You must not smoke, and you must take no drugs whatsoever. It is also a sensible idea to let your doctor know what you are doing, but do not be surprised if the doctor takes it less than seriously. Most doctors are not convinced by the food allergy theory.

Once you have avoided a troublemaker food for several days, you will react much more strongly to it when you do eat it again. This is a good way of double-testing the suspect foods. Even though these foods give you a bad time, do not be surprised if you also long for them—the two together are a sure sign. Once you have isolated the foods to which you are allergic, you should ideally give them up completely. If this is impossible, you could try being "desensitized."

Desensitization

The principle of desensitization is to find a dilution of the food to which the person is allergic that will switch off the allergic reaction to that particular food. Generally speaking, practitioners of clinical ecology prefer MS patients to exercise self-control and avoid the offending foods completely. However, desensitization is a possibility in certain cases.

Rotation Diets

Giving up all foods to which you are allergic is not quite enough. You also need to vary the remaining foods, and make sure that you don't always eat the same thing day in, day out. This is called rotation dieting. Try not to eat one food within three days of having eaten it before. This lessens the chance of developing an allergy to new foods.

Some doctors who practice clinical ecology will allow a prohibited food to be carefully reintroduced after it has been avoided for six to nine months, on the proviso that it is eaten only as part of a rotation diet and not with daily repetition. If you go back to old, addictive eating habits, you could develop masked sensitivity.

OTHER WAYS OF TESTING FOR FOOD ALLERGIES

Around the UK there is now a group of doctors trained in orthodox medicine who have been attracted by certain aspects of alternative medicine. These are the clinical ecologists or doctors trained in nutritional medicine. Because clinical ecology is not taken seriously by the National Health Service (NHS), all of these doctors practice privately. They take the concept of food allergies very seriously and have some novel techniques to test for food and chemical sensitivities. They may use one or a combination of testing techniques.

The testing techniques that they use seem a bit unusual, and it is hard to understand them. One is called the Vega test.

Vega Test

The Vega test works on the principles of bioenergetic regulatory medicine. It looks at the body from an electrical (bioenergetic) sense. It combines aspects of both acupuncture and homeopathy.

The Vega test uses a machine about the size of a hi-fi amplifier. It has buttons, an indicator, and a wire connected to a hand-held electrode and a measuring stylus.

The aim is to place into the machine glass vials containing homeopathic doses of substances (possibly offending foods and chemicals) and find out if these substances are affecting the patient. The patient is given a hand-held cylinder to complete the electrical circuit. As each substance is put into the machine, the operator applies a tiny electrical current via an electrode to a point on the end of a finger or toe. This corresponds with known acupuncture points.

A bleep emits from the machine. If the bleep is low, it indicates that the substance is having a bad effect on the patient's condition. Also, there is a lower reading than normal on the indicator dial. If the sound of the bleep is normal and the reading on the indicator dial is normal, then the person is not allergic to that particular substance. This is a relatively fast and painless way of pinpointing the substances that are toxic to you.

The other new method that seems crazy beyond belief is called applied kinesiology—but it really does seem to work.

Applied Kinesiology

Applied kinesiology also works on the principles of bioenergetic regulatory medicine. It tests the reaction of muscles as a way of detecting food allergies and nutrient imbalances.

The patient is asked to hold in his left hand a glass vial containing a homeopathic dose of a particular substance. The patient will not know what this substance is. (Sometimes the vial is placed on the patient's stomach.) The practitioner will ask the patient to raise his right arm into the air and to resist any pressure put on it by the practitioner.

If the patient is not allergic to the substance in the vial, he will be able to resist the pressure on his right arm from the practitioner. The muscles in his arm will remain strong and of good tone, and he will have no trouble keeping his arm up in the air. The strength in his muscles suggests that he needs the substance.

If the substance given to the patient is toxic to him, however, he will be unable to resist the pressure of the practitioner on his right arm, the arm will feel weak and the muscles lacking in tone, and he will give way under the pressure. The weakness in his muscles suggests that he does not need the substance.

The practitioner of applied kinesiology gives the patient a succession of glass vials, each containing a substance. By putting pressure on the muscles of the raised arm, it is possible to identify those foods and substances to which the patient is allergic.

Many doctors do find applied kinesiology quite unbelievable—more like something out of a magic show than real medicine. Even so, many doctors who were once skeptical have now had to admit that, crazy though it sounds, it does work.

As well as being a way of testing for food allergies, applied kinesiology can also be a treatment. (See Chapter 10 on holistic medicine.)

Cytotoxic Testing

Live white blood cells are exposed to a number of foods and chemicals. If the cells are damaged, this is a sign of sensitivity. The extent to which the cells are damaged gives an indication of the extent of the sensitivity. If there is no damage to the white blood cells, the substance being tested is harmless to that individual.

Intradermal Injection Techniques

This involves injecting tiny amounts of the allergen just beneath the skin surface. A wheal—a small, round bump—appears. If the wheal gets bigger, this suggests an allergy to the substance. If the wheal stays the same size, there is no allergy.

There are other diagnostic techniques to test for food allergies, but those mentioned are the main ones.

Nutritional Profile

Clinical ecologists like first to determine the nutritional profile of each patient by doing various tests. Hair analysis is widely used. Some doctors also use the sweat test, which is a very sophisticated test able to detect the nutritional status of a patient extremely accurately. These tests almost always show that an MS patient is low in zinc.

The nutritional supplements often prescribed by clinical ecologists are covered in detail in the previous chapter. The list includes zinc, iron, selenium, vitamin B_6, vitamin B_{12}. Certain amino acids are also prescribed.

Some doctors find that, once the food allergies and the other ecological problems, such as mercury toxicity or candidiasis, have been treated, the nutrient balance in the body sorts itself out so that supplements are no longer necessary.

Conclusions

From work being done by some doctors both in the UK and the USA, it seems that food allergies should be taken very seriously by anyone with MS. The percentage of people with MS who improve once they avoid the foods to which they are allergic is very impressive.

SUCCESSES WITH EXCLUSION DIETS

The Roger MacDougall Diet

The best known and best publicized people with MS whose lives have changed as a result of identifying their food sensitivities are Roger MacDougall and Alan Greer. At the time of writing, Roger MacDougall is in his seventies. He is in good health with no obvious signs of disability and he travels around the world, writing and lecturing. In 1953, however, he was firmly diagnosed as having MS and showed many of the classic symptoms. Within a few years of diagnosis, his eyesight, legs, fingers, and speech were badly affected. Before long, he was in a wheelchair. Without any medical training (he is a playwright and professor in the University of California's theater department), Roger MacDougall decided to set about finding ways of treating his degenerative condition.

By a mixture of inspiration, guesswork, research, shots in the dark, and borrowing from other dietary regimens for MS, Roger MacDougall devised his own diet for MS. It began as just a gluten-free diet but has evolved to exclude sugar and dairy products. It is also now high in polyunsaturated fats and low in saturated fats, and it has a long list of vitamin, mineral, trace element, and other supplements.

In his own case, Roger MacDougall has experienced an impressive recovery that anyone can witness for themselves. He boasts of being able to leap not just up the stairs two at a time, but *down* the stairs two at a time as well. Anyone with MS will appreciate that this is indeed some feat.

Roger MacDougall's diet used to be known as the "gluten-free diet" when it was first devised, but this is now a serious misnomer. Over the years, Roger MacDougall has moved with the times, and his original diet has evolved quite considerably. It has four equally important elements:

1. no gluten
2. low sugar and no refined sugar

3. low milk products/high polyunsaturates
4. supplements of vitamins, minerals, and trace elements

MacDougall first singled out gluten, which is the elastic-type component in dough. In celiac disease, the sufferer is allergic to gluten. MacDougall thought that this could also be happening in MS. He linked MS with celiac disease because in celiac disease the patient cannot assimilate fats. However, once wheat, barley, oats, and rye are removed totally from the diet, fats can be taken into the body without any problem. MacDougall suggests that foods containing gluten "damage the lining of the small intestine in such a way that the nutrients required to keep renewing the myelin sheath are prevented from reaching the bloodstream."

In celiac disease, the mucosal lining of the bowel is damaged so nutrients cannot be absorbed properly. MacDougall wondered if people with MS were experiencing something similar.

Sugar was excluded because of its role in causing hypoglycemia, which can happen with MS. As for dairy products, their connection with the geographical distribution of MS was well known, and MS shows the same world distribution as cardiovascular disease. The vitamins, minerals, trace elements, and other supplements make up for all of the nutrients you would be lacking if you gave up all cereals and dairy products.

Gluten

Excluding gluten means excluding all foods containing wheat, barley, oats, and rye. This wipes out nearly all bread, cakes, biscuits, crispbreads, pasta, many breakfast cereals, and vast numbers of canned and processed foods—look on the labels.

Recently, researchers from the National Institute of Mental Health in Washington found that gluten gives rise to substances called opioids in the gut. Some people cannot digest these, and researchers have found that they may block the conversion of dihomo-gamma-linolenic acid to series 1 prostaglandins.

An Australian, Dr. R. Shatin from Melbourne, has suggested that demyelination of the nerve sheaths is secondary to an intolerance for gluten in the small intestine. He also put forward the hypothesis that the high rate of MS in Canada, Scotland, and Western Ireland may be due to the predominant use of Canadian wheat, which has the highest content of gluten of any in the world.

The cereals that you can eat after you have excluded gluten are rice, maize (corn), and millet. You can safely use products such as rice flour, cornmeal, breakfast cereals made with rice and corn (no added sugar), sago, and tapioca. Of course, these would only be OK if you were not allergic to any of them. (It is quite common to be allergic to corn.)

Sugar

This means eating nothing made from refined sugar or any product containing it, e.g., jams, marmalades, cakes, cookies, canned fruit, sweets, chocolate, ice cream, most drinks, processed foods, etc. For sweetness, you could eat honey, raw Barbados sugar (not Demerara), raw sugar chocolate, fructose, all fresh and dried fruits. (Make sure you are not allergic to sugar, though.)

Fat

Cut out butter, cream, full-cream milk, and high fat cheeses. Do not eat fatty meats like bacon, pork, duck, or goose or processed meats like sausages.

Use only polyunsaturated margarine. (Watch out for whey, which is a milk product.) For cooking and salad dressing, use sunflower seed oil or safflower seed oil. You can use small quantities of skimmed milk, low fat cottage cheese, low fat yogurt, and eggs.

Organ meats like liver, kidneys, tongue, sweetbreads, and brain can all be eaten. So can free-range animals such as venison, rabbit, and poultry. *Lean* cuts of meat like beef or pork are OK.

Drinks

Many drinks contain gluten, sugar, or both. Give up ale, beer, whiskey, gin, instant coffee, hot cocoa, malted drinks, fizzy drinks, etc. Instead, drink natural sugar-free fruit and vegetable juices, tea, decaffeinated coffee, cider, and mineral waters.

Other Foods

All other foods not on the exclusion list are OK to eat, e.g., all vegetables and legumes, seeds, nuts, all fish, all herbs, and spices and condiments. (Use only natural essences and flavorings.)

These are permitted on the Roger MacDougall diet because none of these things contain gluten, sugar, or saturated fat. If you believe in the principle of food allergy, however, it would be possible for you to be allergic to any of the above, e.g., tomatoes, bananas, or peanuts.

Supplements of Vitamins, Minerals, Trace Elements

Supplements are necessary because cutting out so many grains and dairy products also cuts out many other nutrients. The vitamins, minerals, and trace elements must be replaced. Roger MacDougall's list of supplements is remarkably similar to the list described in the previous chapters.

Vitamins: B vitamins choline bitartrate, vitamin B_1, vitamin B_2, vitamin B_6, folic acid, inositol, nicotinamide, and pantothenic acid; vitamin C, and vitamin E
Lipids: lecithin, evening primrose oil
Minerals and trace elements: magnesium, zinc, copper, iron, selenium

Roger MacDougall has quite a considerable following and receives heartening letters from people who have followed his dietary guidelines and improved. His diet excludes a number of foods, any one (or more) of which could be causing allergy problems. Indeed, the Roger MacDougall diet may be working in so many people because the excluded foods include some of the most common allergic foods.

Rather than go on such a rigid diet, another approach would be to test yourself first for food allergies. It would be a pity to give up *all* grains if you were only allergic to, say, wheat.

Cutting down—or cutting out—sugar is good advice, but there are two distinct types of sugar—cane and beet. If you get yourself tested, you may find you are allergic to one but not the other.

It's a similar story with milk—cutting down on full-cream milk is good advice. However, milk is the most common allergic food for people with MS. If you tested positive for milk allergy, it would not help to continue taking any kind of milk at all, even skimmed milk or low fat yogurts or cheeses.*

The Rita Greer Diet

The other well-publicized exclusion diet with a successful outcome is the Rita Greer diet. Rita Greer began experimenting with foods for her husband Alan when he was severely disabled and doctors had written him off as a hopeless case. Her first breakthrough was when she accidentally discovered that Alan felt better on a diet that totally excluded meat—something she was forced to do through sheer poverty. From that, it was a short step to discover that he reacted badly to eggs and cheese and all saturated fat. Rita also decided to follow the principles of the gluten-free diet and cut out everything made with wheat, barley, oats, and rye.

By this time (early 1970s), sunflower seed oil was gaining popularity as a supplement for MS patients. So Rita began by giving her husband daily doses of sunflower seed oil. As soon as Naudicelle became available, she replaced sunflower seed oil with these capsules of evening primrose oil.

With much trial and error, hard work, study of nutrition, and the creativity that goes with being a gifted artist, Rita eventually came up with a diet that suited Alan's body perfectly. She kept him on this basically vegan diet for about four years, during which time he made gigantic improvements to the point where the wheelchair and walking aids were banished with the bedpans to the lumber room. His regeneration was so startling that some doctors were doubtful that he had ever had MS at all, as

---

*For full details of Roger McDougall's diet and supplements, contact Regenics Ltd, 209 Blackburn Road, Wheelton, Chorley, Lancs. PR6 8EP, England. Tel: 0254-830122.

his improved condition did not tally with his medical notes. There is no doubt, however, that Alan Greer did and does have MS. It is just that he no longer eats the foods that were having a toxic effect on him.

Rita Greer had an easy task finding out which foods made Alan worse—he was sick if he ate something to which he was allergic. This is a very dramatic response, and allergic reactions are usually more subtle.

The list of foods to which Alan was allergic may not be the same list for anyone else with MS. His list of allergic foods was as follows:

butter, cheese, milk, cream, yogurt, lard, eggs, meat, fatty fish like herring and tuna, shellfish
wheat, barley, oats, rye, and everything made with them (such as bread, pasta, biscuits, cakes, breakfast cereals, custard powder)
cane sugar, honey, jam, molasses, sweets, chocolate
drinking chocolate, malted drinks, cocoa, coffee, strong tea, squashes, cordials, spirits, alcoholic drinks
canned fruit, canned vegetables, bananas, avocados, peanuts, brazil nuts, hazelnuts, chestnuts
packaged, canned, and processed foods, semolina, bouillon cubes, spreads and dips

Alan also gave up smoking. He took supplements of evening primrose oil, multi-vitamin and mineral tablets, and vitamin B_{12} (essential for non–meat eaters). Even though he excluded many foods, this still left him with a wide choice, especially of fruits and vegetables and white fish. However, there is no guarantee that the fruits and vegetables that were perfectly OK for Alan Greer would not cause reactions in someone else with MS.

The conclusion from both the Roger MacDougall diet and the Rita Greer diet is to get yourself tested for your own personal food allergies before copying what someone else did. What worked for them might not work for you, and it would be foolish to go on these difficult diets if they are not tailor-made for your needs.

10

Holistic Medicine

Many therapies that come under the broad heading of holistic or alternative medicine can be very helpful in MS. These include not only the well-established therapies such as acupuncture, osteopathy, and homeopathy, but also the newer ones such as aromatherapy, applied kinesiology, electromagnetic crystal therapy, and reflexology.

Many of the holistic therapies share some of the concepts of the ancient Eastern systems of medicine in which balance is synonymous with good health. Good health is harmony: a balance between opposing forces, between yin and yang, or between acid and alkaline.

Harmony also involves much more than just a biochemical balance. As in the traditional Eastern forms of medicine, it also means right life, wisdom and love, right fellowship, meditation, healthy eating, and exercise.

No matter what therapy you are talking about, any kind of alternative therapy is likely to be holistic in its approach. Unlike the orthodox doctor, the alternative therapist will attempt to treat you as a whole person—mind, body, and spirit—and not just treat the diseased part. This holistic approach also extends to the treatment itself, which can encompass every aspect of a person's life and not just their physical symptoms.

In fact, the whole approach of all alternative therapies is radically different from orthodox medicine. By and large, alternative practitioners are not very interested in giving diseases labels such as multiple sclerosis or arthritis. Broadly, they tend to view disease as a loss of balance in the body, brought about by an imbalanced lifestyle and thought patterns.

These practitioners also tend to believe that, with help, the body can be brought back into balance and that good health can be regained. They generally do not go along with the concept of "incurable" diseases. Although none would claim to "cure" MS, many do say that the condition can be stabilized and that the downward spiral can be stopped or even reversed.

Orthodox medicine diagnoses symptoms and tries to find ways of suppressing those symptoms, usually through drugs. By contrast, holistic therapists aim not to suppress symptoms, but to get to the root cause or causes of the symptoms and to treat those root causes instead.

The general starting point with alternative medicine is the conviction that the body has innate powers to heal itself given the right conditions. The task of any alternative therapist is to help bring about the right conditions so the body can get on with the business of healing itself.

The mistake some patients make is to view a particular alternative therapy as just a technique. This is a very conventional, passive view of medicine. If you want any kind of holistic therapy to be helpful, you have to be an active participant in the healing process and not just a passive recipient who has something done to you.

Before you see any holistic practitioner (which includes some trained doctors), you should be psychologically prepared to change many aspects of your life fundamentally. The therapy itself is likely to be only one part of a holistic treatment program, which may involve quite dramatic changes in diet, lifestyle, exercise, and thought patterns.

The whole attitude of holistic medicine transforms your way of thinking and makes you think seriously about how *you* came to have MS. You may well, with the help of the therapist, discover aspects of your old lifestyle that must be changed now if you want to get better and not worse.

Getting involved in alternative medicine may well mean making radical changes to your lifestyle, how you eat, what you eat, what you drink, and the way you think. The approach of alternative medicine is very positive and hopeful, as you no longer classify yourself in the orthodox mode of being someone with an incurable illness. Instead, you see yourself as someone who is making profound changes to help regain health.

IS ALTERNATIVE THERAPY EFFECTIVE?

There are claims from many holistic therapists that what they do can help MS patients. They never use the word "cure," as this is not the way they think. It is difficult to be precise about to what extent they can be effective. This differs from case to case. It is always hard to turn the clock back and reverse existing damage. Some already-disabled people may feel increased well being as a result of seeing a holistic practitioner, and someone with only mild MS symptoms may find that these symptoms do go away with treatment. Everyone, no matter what their degree of the disease, should experience a greater sense of well-being as a result of treatment in the chosen therapy, together with some lifestyle changes.

WHAT ALTERNATIVE THERAPY?

I do not intend to go into detail about all of the various alternative or holistic therapies—how they work and what they do. There are several good books that do that. An excellent one is *The Natural Family Doctor*, edited by Dr. Andrew Stanway (Century). Which therapy, or therapies, you choose may depend on what appeals to you most, or which one has been recommended to you, or what is available in your area. Many therapists are trying to achieve the same ends by different means.

I had good personal experiences with several therapies, and they may have played a part in stabilizing my condition. These are, specifically, acupuncture, osteopathy, hydrotherapy, herbalism, applied kinesiology, massage, reflexology, and electromagnetic crystal therapy. Nearly all of the alternative therapies have been used to treat patients with multiple sclerosis. These are (in no particular order):

homeopathy
herbalism
aromatherapy
naturopathy
hydrotherapy
osteopathy
cranial osteopathy
chiropractic
massage

applied kinesiology
reflexology
acupuncture
shiatsu
Alexander technique
healing
meditation (see also the chapter on yoga)
electromagnetic crystal therapy

Quite often, if you see one therapist, he or she may refer you to another therapy or therapies if you could benefit from another approach as well.

I believe that it is worth getting involved in the whole field of holistic medicine, at the very least because it transforms your attitudes and your lifestyle to healthier ones. At the very best, it can improve your health.

11

Mercury in Dental Fillings

IS MS A REACTION TO ENVIRONMENTAL TOXINS?

Some doctors working in the field of environmental medicine believe that degenerative diseases such as multiple sclerosis are a sort of slow poisoning of the system. Everyday things in our environment that are harmless to most people prove to be toxic to some susceptible people. The people who are susceptible to environmental toxins seem to have a poorer ability to adapt than others. Case histories of patients who have been treated in this field show that, if they are exposed to certain environmental toxins, their symptoms get worse but, when those toxins are taken away, the symptoms get better.

Food has already been discussed in some detail. The other things that can be toxic to people with MS are a whole range of chemicals found in our everyday lives and also certain metals. Chemicals are discussed in the next chapter.

Of all the metals that can be toxic to someone with MS, mercury is probably the worst. Mercury is a toxic metal, yet it has been used in amalgam dental fillings for more than a century. Recently, there has been growing concern that some of this mercury could be seeping into the body, causing serious health problems, sometimes including neurological symptoms.

The people who have dared to raise their voices against mercury in dental fillings are a few dentists, nutritionists, and a handful of doctors in both the USA and the UK. They are up against the majority of the dental and medical establishment, who insist that the mercury in fillings is safe and who take the view that linking MS symptoms to the mercury in your fillings is unproven and irresponsible. This heated controversy is still being argued in the dental and medical literature.

THE CASE AGAINST MERCURY

Mercury is one of the most toxic poisons known to humans. When it was first used as a component in fillings, dentists thought it was safe because it was used together with other metals.

What Fillings Are Made Of

Pure mercury (also known as quicksilver) is mixed with particles of silver, copper, and tin to form a putty-like mix. This mix— or amalgam—is placed in the tooth. The mercury hardens and holds these particles together.

Mercury Can Get into the Body

Because mercury was mixed with these other metals, it was thought to be stable, but mercury in amalgam fillings is not stable. Mercury, in a variety of forms, can get into the body. It can leak into the tooth or gum; you can swallow it with saliva; you can breathe it in.

Over the years, mercury seeps from fillings in minute amounts. How much mercury seeps out depends on how much dental plaque there is, the pH (acid/alkaline balance) inside the mouth, how old the fillings are, how many fillings you have, how hard you chew, what food you eat, your individual body chemistry, and so on.

As well as the chronic low level exposure, every day, for years on end, there is also acute exposure to mercury vapor when you are having a filling put in or taken out. Elemental mercury gives off a vapor when it is agitated, compressed, heated, or exposed to air at normal temperature. It is easy to breathe this vapor in. It goes through the thin bony plates at the top of the mouth, into the sinuses, into the orbit of the eye, and the chambers of the inner ear where the body's balancing mechanism is situated. It also gets into the brain, which is so near the top of the mouth. It also goes into the temporomandibular joint, which controls the functions of the jaw. Mercury vapor also gets into the lungs.

Various biological processes inside the body transform mercury vapor into methyl mercury, which is one hundred times more toxic than mercury vapor. Mercury vapor can mix with food. When it gets into the stomach, mercury can react with hydrochloric acid, resulting in the formation of mercuric chloride. This can create a shortage of hydrochloric acid, which means that food cannot be digested properly.

Fillings Provide a Continuous Source of Mercury

Even though your body will be excreting mercury (which is measurable), some mercury will remain in your system. How much mercury is there, where exactly it is, and what it is doing to you are far less easy to measure.

If you have several fillings in your mouth, you have a continuous source of mercury. This means that, in the course of a life span, mercury will be accumulated in almost every organ.

Research has shown that amalgam fillings do not remain the same as the day they were put in and that there is a substantial loss of mercury. In the USA, researchers found an astonishingly high loss of mercury compared with the original filling. What this means is that you could have ingested anything between 30 and 560 mg of mercury particles or vapor over the years, depending on the number of fillings you have. On a day-to-day basis, this is a very small amount of mercury, but even tiny amounts of mercury can be damaging.

Fillings will corrode in time. This corrosion is partly because fillings are subjected to all of the chemicals put into the mouth, both from food and drink and those produced by your own body. The corrosion is also partly due to electrical activity.

Mercury from corroded amalgam fillings can get into the body. You can inhale the vapor, or swallow or convert the particles that result from corrosion.

Your Mouth Is Like an Electrical Generator

If you have more than one kind of metal in your mouth, then you have electricity in your mouth. This is because all metals are reservoirs of energy called electrons. If electrons can flow through some kind of conductor, then you have an electrical current. Saliva is an electrolyte (an aqueous solution with metal ions capable of transporting an electrical current).

This electrical activity can cause corrosion of fillings. It can also affect the function of cranial nerves, which in itself can affect any system in the body.

Where Does Mercury inside Your Body Go?

Mercury can go everywhere—it is able to travel all over the body, upsetting intricate processes. Primarily, mercury affects the central nervous system. Mercury can inactivate the lymphocytes and alter the ratio between T-suppressor and T-helper cells.

Mercury can also accumulate in the kidneys, heart muscle, lungs, liver, brain, and red blood cells. Other areas where mercury can be stored are the thyroid gland, pituitary gland, adrenal glands, spleen, testes, bone marrow, and intestinal wall. Mercury can get through the blood-brain barrier and enter the nerve cells from the blood, destroying nerve tissue as it does so.

What Damage Does Mercury Do?

Most people are not affected by the mercury in their fillings—not overtly, anyway. Some people are, however.

As mercury is capable of damaging many tissues and organs, thereby disturbing their normal functions, it is not surprising that the list of symptoms that can be caused by mercury poisoning is very long. A general list includes bleeding gums, increased salivation, a sour-metallic taste, facial paralysis, irregular heartbeat, depression, strong pains in the left part of chest, retinal bleeding, dim vision, uncontrollable eye movement, irritability, vertigo, headaches, joint pains, pains in the lower back, stress intolerance, decreased sexual activity, and Bell's palsy.

Specifically neurological symptoms include mild tremor, ataxia (lack of muscle coordination and irregular movement), sensory loss, visual problems, fatigue, numbness and tingling of hands, feet, or lips, muscle weakness progressing to paralysis, speech disorders, and general central nervous system dysfunctions.

Mercury has a devastating effect on the body's immune system, particularly on the T cells, which have a vital part to play in cell-mediated immunity. This means that mercury can alter the body's defense mechanisms against infection and disease and also make people more prone to allergy. In addition, mercury may cause vascular damage to the brain and spinal cord. MS is now considered by many to be primarily a vascular disorder.

MERCURY IN FILLINGS AND MULTIPLE SCLEROSIS

Is multiple sclerosis mercury poisoning? Do some of the neurological symptoms from mercury poisoning mimic multiple sclerosis? Are people with MS especially sensitive to mercury? Or does mercury simply enhance MS symptoms?

No one knows for sure whether mercury triggers MS, or exacerbates MS, or mimics MS. However, if it has triggered MS, this does not mean you can cure the patient by removing the mercury, but you can improve the symptoms by doing so.

In both the UK and the USA, there have been several documented cases of people who were told that they had MS, had their fillings removed, and then recovered from their "MS" symptoms. In his book about mercury amalgam dental fillings, *The Toxic Time Bomb* (Thorsons), author Sam Ziff described some such cases, and the British media have also highlighted a few cases. Did these people really have MS? Or did their symptoms just seem like MS? Or was their MS made worse by the mercury poisoning? The general view among the doctors and dentists who believe that there is a connection between mercury and MS is that mercury can exacerbate MS symptoms or cause symptoms that mimic MS, but that it does *not* actually *cause* MS. They believe that there is already a predisposition to MS that was there before any fillings were put in.

In some cases, it seems that the neurological symptoms mimic multiple sclerosis and that therefore the diagnosis of MS is a mistaken one. London dentist Vicky Lee says,

> Many patients with MS have been diagnosed only on clinical symptoms, and these symptoms may be identical with heavy metal poisoning—in particular mercury poisoning with symptoms such as tremor, ataxia, irritability, fatigue, cold sweats, frequent urination and eye symptoms.

The Hypothesis that Mercury Poisoning Leads to MS

However, there are some people who believe that mercury in fillings *is* a cause of MS. In 1983, an article entitled "Epidemiology, Etiology, and Prevention of Multiple Sclerosis" written by Theodore H. Ingalls, M.D., of the Epidemiology Study Center in Framingham, Massachusetts, was published in the *Journal of Forensic Medicine and Pathology* (vol. 4, number 1, March 1983). It began:

> Slow, retrograde seepage of ionic mercury from root canal or . . . amalgam fillings inserted many years previously, recurrent caries and corrosion around filling edges, and the oxidizing effect of the purulent response may lead to Multiple Sclerosis in middle age.

Dr. Ingalls, himself an MS sufferer, goes on to say that the world map of MS could be explained by the greater incidence of dental caries in the parts of the world where MS is high and the lower incidence of dental caries in those parts of the world where MS is low. Obviously, the more dental caries there are, the more fillings there are. He suggests that perhaps dental caries are a precursor of MS. As well as mercury, Dr. Ingalls thinks that lead may be involved in MS.

> Clinical and epidemiologic data also suggest that a second heavy metal, lead, may operate almost interchangeably with mercury.

Possibly, cases of unilateral (one side only) MS derive from mercury amalgam fillings in teeth, whereas the generalized disease may result from ingestion or inhalation of volatile mercury or exhaust fumes of lead additives to gasoline (petrol).

Dr. Ingalls also argues that heavy metal poisoning may be coming from other sources apart from tooth fillings.

Heavy Metal Poisoning from Farming and Industrial Techniques

Certain fungicides and weedkillers contain mercury. Perhaps this is a factor that might help explain why MS is higher in farming than fishing areas. Mercury is also found in some industrial germicides.

SHOULD YOU HAVE YOUR FILLINGS REMOVED?

This question is not as simple as it seems. Not everyone with MS is necessarily reacting to the mercury in their fillings. No one has been taking reliable statistics, but it seems that more than half of those people with MS who have been tested for mercury sensitivity show positive results. If you are sensitive to mercury, you should consider having your fillings out. It would not be worth having your fillings taken out if you show no sensitivity to mercury.

There are certain tests that can indicate whether you are hypersensitive to mercury. One, using an electrical meter, measures the electrical activity in the mouth. The other methods are the Vega test and applied kinesiology (see the chapter on food allergies). To have these tests, you would have to consult a private dentist or a clinical ecologist.

Dangers in the Removal of Fillings

The removal of fillings is not a simple matter, and there are dangers in the procedure. The danger with removing fillings is that mercury vapor is released into the air. There seems to be little disagreement that the highest levels of mercury vapor are reached during the insertion and removal of amalgam, with a potential danger to both the patient and the dental practitioner. Some dentists are willing to place a full-mouth rubber dam in the mouth, which prevents mercury vapor from escaping. As an extra precaution, they might take out only a few fillings at a time instead of several or even all of them. This would make the removal of a large number of fillings a lengthy procedure as well as an expensive one.

However, there is no doubt that some people with MS have shown dramatic improvement after their fillings have been removed. Along with the more publicized cases of people with MS whose symptoms have disappeared after the removal of their fillings, there are also cases where the MS has worsened after a full-scale removal of fillings.

The first thing to do is to find a sympathetic dentist, get yourself tested, and then follow his or her advice. Even those dentists who believe that there is an overwhelming connection between mercury in your fillings and MS may think it is better to leave them alone if you show no sensitivity to mercury, as improvements can be astounding. It is fair to say that the removal of fillings *may* help in MS, rather than *will* help.

OTHER ASPECTS OF MULTIPLE SCLEROSIS AND DENTISTRY

Some holistic doctors have found that people with MS have problems with their temporomandibular joint. This is a hinge joint in the jaw that articulates the mandible and the temporal bones. With a temporomandibular joint problem, the teeth are out of alignment. A cranial osteopath should be able to correct this. Some people with MS have reported that once their temporomandibular joint problem was corrected by a skilled cranial osteopath, there was an improvement in other MS symptoms.

MERCURY AND MICRONUTRIENTS

Many people with MS are low in zinc, manganese, chromium, selenium, and other trace elements. Of these, the most important is zinc (see Chapter 8). If you were to weigh the amount of mercury being placed in a large filling, there might be as much as 1 gram of mercury alone. There is potentially enough mercury in the mouth to interfere with the micronutrients of the body.

The amount of mercury released during the placement and removal of an amalgam filling is certainly enough to unbalance the very tiny amounts of micronutrients even in a healthy person, at least for a short time.

When the body is short of essential micronutrients, it has a greater chance of being susceptible to mercury poisoning. If there is a shortage of zinc and selenium, mercury cannot bind to zinc/selenium protein complexes. So mercury can rampage freely around the body, locked in because the mechanism for its removal is not there. The body may be attempting to rid itself of mercury through the bile and sweat, but in fact may be reabsorbing mercury in the colon and through the skin, particularly if someone is not very physically active, cannot wash himself daily, and is constipated.

CAN YOU DETOXIFY YOURSELF OF MERCURY WITHOUT HAVING ALL YOUR FILLINGS REMOVED?

Nutritional methods on their own will not be sufficient to detoxify the body of mercury, although they will help. If you have all the tests and you do show a sensitivity to mercury, then it is probably best to have your fillings taken out. Even after you have done this, however, there will still be mercury left in your body. The removal of fillings will get rid of about 50 percent of the mercury, but that still leaves the other 50 percent to be eliminated.

You should follow up the removal of fillings with nutritional methods. Even if you don't show any sensitivity to mercury and don't have your fillings removed, it would be a good idea to follow the same nutritional program, which is designed to escort toxins out of the body. It is possible that, if your nutrition is optimal, you can reverse a sensitivity to mercury shown in the tests mentioned.

Oral Chelation Therapy

The nutritional method that can help detoxify the body is called "oral chelation therapy." Chelation simply means latching on to something else. As well as helping to detoxify the body, oral chelation therapy is a way of replacing essential nutrients that may be inactivated by low level, chronic exposure to mercury.

Find a multivitamin and mineral product that also contains the amino acids cysteine and methionine. These have something called sulfhydryl groups. These are particularly effective at latching on to toxic minerals such as lead or mercury. Once this latching-on process has happened, vitamin C (1 gram three times daily) will help to excrete these toxic metals from the body.

Sulfhydryl groups are also present in onions and garlic. These are also valuable in detoxifying the body. However, they should be avoided if you are on homoeopathic remedies, as they act as an antidote.

Information about the following nutrients that help to detoxify the body comes from *The Toxic Time Bomb*, written by Sam Ziff and published by Thorsons Publishing Group.

Cysteine

The amino acid cysteine has a specific affinity for mercury and will bind with it, allowing excretion of it from the body. Vitamin C must be taken with cysteine at a ratio of 3:1. (Cysteine is in Health Insurance Plus—see above.)

Glutathione

Glutathione is composed of the amino acids cysteine, glutamic acid, and glycine and serves as a storage and transport vehicle for cysteine. Glutathione is a water-soluble anti-oxidant and free radical scavenger and acts as a detoxicant against heavy metal toxins. It works with vitamins C and E, adding to their roles as anti-oxidants. The suggested dose is 50 mg twice daily.

Vitamin C and Vitamin E

These are important agents against mercury because mercury is known to cause free radicals in the body, and these vitamins scavenge and mop up free radicals. Research papers show that vitamin E can reduce the toxic effects of mercury. In laboratory tests, vitamin E was able to reduce the chromosomal breakage caused by mercury. The suggested dose of vitamin C is 1,000 to 3,000 mg, and that of vitamin E is 100 to 400 i.u.

Selenium and Molybdenum

Some studies have shown that selenium and molybdenum can reduce the toxic effects of mercury. Do not exceed 200 μg of selenium a day, as it can be toxic.

Zinc

Mercury can displace zinc in the body, yet zinc is a vital trace element that latches on to mercury and escorts it out of the body. The suggested dose is 20 to 50 mg a day.

Magnesium

Mercury can inhibit various enzyme systems in the body by inhibiting the activity of magnesium. The suggested dose is 100 to 200 mg per day. Be careful of creating an imbalance between magnesium and calcium. If necessary, take calcium supplements or Dolomite, a mixture of calcium and magnesium carbonates.

Vitamin B_6

Vitamin B_6 is involved in how the body handles the detoxification of mercury. The suggested dose is 50 to 200 mg daily.

Rutin

Rutin is one of the bioflavenoid family. It seems to have a specificity for binding to and helping to remove mercury from the body.

Calcium Pantothenate or Pantothenic Acid

The physiologically active form of pantothenic acid is co-enzyme A. Mercury can inhibit or suppress co-enzyme A, which is also a co-factor involved in adrenal function. Pantothenic acid should be taken if fillings are removed, as this is an additional stress to the body. The dose is 100 to 400 mg daily.

Vitamin B_1 (Thiamine)

Thiamine is important in the decarboxylation process of cellular respiration. There is a critical step at the entrance into the aerobic oxidation cycle. This step involves co-enzyme A. Co-enzyme A carries fatty acids to the membranes of the mitochondria and hands them over to the amino acid carnitine, which crosses the inner membrane of the mitochondria. Carnitine then hands over the fatty acids to another molecule of co-enzyme A. The mitochondria are the power centers of each cell. It is in the mitochondria that glucose and fatty acids are oxidized to generate the energy that powers us. Co-enzyme A contains a sulfhydryl group (SH). These SH groups are susceptible to being inactivated by mercury and so unable to produce acetyl-co-enzyme A.

Adding thiamine helps to repair the impaired area of the metabolic cycle. The limited amounts of co-enzyme A still available are used more efficiently.

The dose of thiamine is 50 mg morning and evening. It should be taken in a B complex tablet.

Acidophilus

Acidophilus is a friendly bacteria found in live yogurt, which goes to make up intestinal flora. The intestinal flora may play a significant part in determining the excretion rate of mercury.

Candida (see Chapter 9)

There is a relationship betwen candidiasis and mercury. There seems to be a connection between the presence of amalgam and the body's ability to cope with the yeast *Candida albicans*. *Candida* is considered normal flora, but when the body's immune mechanisms are impaired, *Candida* can increase until it produces disease-like symptoms. If you are sensitive to mercury, *Candida* organisms are resistant to treatment. Once you get rid of mercury, however, candidiasis is more amenable to treatment.

12

Chemicals and Other Environmental Toxins

The list of chemicals and other environmental toxins that could affect someone with MS is very long indeed. It includes many of the things that you probably take for granted in your everyday life, such as aerosol sprays, tap water, and even chipboard. More obvious toxins include lead from car exhaust fumes and—worse—diesel fumes. And, of course, cigarette smoke.

Many of these things, such as cosmetics made from coal tar or food with artificial coloring, you may have used for several years. So why do they seem to be having a bad effect on you now? This could be because of toxic overload.

TOXIC OVERLOAD

Some people are better able to adapt to new stresses than others. The theory of the general adaptation syndrome comes originally from Dr. Theron Randolph, the founding father of clinical ecology in the USA.

Roughly, the theory goes like this: The syndrome begins with repeated, occasional exposure to any irritant substance. At a certain level of exposure, the person has a rejection response, or "alarm" response. The alarm response will happen any time the person is exposed to the substance, as long as this exposure happens only now and again.

However, if the exposure happens more than occasionally (i.e., frequently or all the time), the response is different. The person seems to be adapted to the substance. This is the "resistance" phase.

This apparent adaptation, however, is not a genuine adaptation at all. What in fact is going on is that the body is making a huge internal effort to cope with the stresses of the substance.

The body makes much larger quantities than usual of hormones such as cortisone and epinephrine. These hormones in the blood can give you a boost of energy and a feeling of well-being, but it is not long-lived because, after a short time, these hormones are spent.

When this happens, the person may seek out the substance, like an addict. If this addiction is not satisfied, the adaptation breaks down. When this happens, the reaction to the substance becomes the alarm response again, but in a more dramatic form.

The phase when the body's adaptive ability breaks down is called the "exhaustion" phase. The affected person may feel ill or irritable all the time. The way out of this is to withdraw the offending substance from the person. At first, this may have the effect of making him or her more ill, but there is no other way to get the whole system back on an even keel.

A wide range of symptoms can be explained by this general adaptation syndrome. Its effects extend into behavior, thinking, and personality. All of these reactions can be caused by foods, chemicals, or metals.

It could be argued that anyone with MS has already reached the exhaustion phase. If you can identify which things are causing *your* toxic overload and if you can then remove these things from your life, there is the chance of getting better instead of getting worse.

Two very helpful books that go into this subject in great detail are *Chemical Children* by Dr. Peter Mansfield and Dr. Jean Monro (Century paperbacks, 1987), and *Clinical Ecology* by Dr. George T. Lewith and Dr. Julian N. Kenyon (Thorsons, 1985).

CHEMICALS IN FOODS

Be aware of chemicals in foods. Read labels like a hawk when you go shopping. With a new awareness, you can totally avoid chemicals in foods.

Unnatural, degraded, processed food may be a cause of de-

Unnatural, degraded, processed food may be a cause of degenerative diseases, of which MS is one. It is only in this century that a whole generation has grown up with eating food that has been adulterated.

Chemical fertilizers, pesticides, and insecticides assault fruit, vegetables, and crops while they are growing. Steroids and antibiotics are given to intensively reared livestock.

In the manufacturing process, a whole range of additives may be added to foods, including artificial colorings, flavorings, and preservatives. In the last few years the public has been alerted to the additives in manufactured foods, and there has been a link made between certain additives in foods and hyperactivity in children. However, the additives in foods may also be affecting people who have MS. Chemicals that are taken in food and drink (or breathed in) can soon produce allergic-type responses.

Even food that you think looks perfectly "natural" may have been polluted before it reached you, the consumer. In fact, the more perfect the specimen of fruit or vegetable, the more suspicious of it you should be. Only fruit and vegetables that have been successfully protected (by chemicals) will be in "perfect" condition by the time they reach the supermarket or produce stand.

How to Avoid Chemicals in Foods

Do not buy anything that is processed. All junk food is out. Whenever you buy anything in a can or a packet, at least read the label. If there are any additives, preservatives, colorings, flavorings—don't buy it.

As a rule, always try to buy pure, fresh things instead of processed foods. The fresher the food, the more "alive" it is. Frozen food will have lost some of its goodness and may have coloring in it, such as the bright green used on frozen peas.

If you can, switch to organic food. It is getting easier all the time to find places that sell organic food—not just organically grown fruit and vegetables, but also meat, poultry, bread, dried produce, etc., which are free of all chemicals.

CHEMICALS IN EVERYDAY LIFE

The most dangerous place to find chemicals that could affect your health is your own home. The chances are that every single room in your home will have things in it to which you could be reacting badly. Here are just some of the culprits.

- *Tap water* contains chlorine, nitrates, and possibly fluoride and polyphosphates.
- *Aerosol sprays*, such as furniture polish, air freshener, fly spray, perfume, deodorant, etc., all use a liquid propellant. When you press the button, a spray of fine droplets of this propellant squirts out under the pressure of the gas in the can. This propellant liquid evaporates, leaving fine particles of the chemical in the air. The technical name for this kind of gas is halocarbon (carbon compounds that contain chlorine, fluorine, or bromine).
- *Fumes from gas boiler*, stove, or fires if ventilation is bad.
- *Chipboard and foam in furniture* give off a type of gas called formaldehyde. Formaldehyde is also found in other common items in the home, such as the combustion products of natural gas, tobacco smoke, glossy magazines and books, and newspapers.

There is a hypothesis that people with MS are grossly contaminated with formaldehyde. Mr. R. C. Baskerville has written lengthy papers on the topic but was denied a grant from any of the MS associations to do further research. He can be contacted at

Baskerville Technical Services
1 Russell Close
Stevenage, SG2 8PB, UK

Other noxious chemicals in the home include

- plastics (even though you can't see it, they give off a gas)
- chemicals in cleaning agents, insect killers, weed killers, etc.
- synthetic carpets and fabrics (which are treated with insecticide in the manufacturing process)

- all solvents—glues, typewriter correcting fluid, nail polish, nail polish remover, dry cleaning fluid, etc., and gloss paint
- cosmetics and toiletries made from coal tar products
- cosmetics and toiletries made with chemical colorants (watch out for brightly colored bath salts, colored toilet paper, etc.)
- toothpaste containing fluoride and coloring (the adverse effects of fluoride include interference with a wide range of metabolic enzymes)

These chemicals can be inhaled through the airways, absorbed through the skin, or ingested. For example, watch out for dishwashing liquid on plates that have not been rinsed properly— the detergent can affect the stomach lining.

Unless you are obviously sensitive to these chemicals (for example, sneezing terribly if someone uses aerosol hair spray), you may not be aware that the gases given off by some of these products may be affecting you. As well as halocarbon vapor from all sorts of aerosols, the same sort of gas comes from solvents used in cosmetics, glues, stain removers, cleaning fluids, etc. Other gases that are given off from common household products are acetone and ether. All of these gases dissolve into the air completely, leaving no haze. Although you can't see them, they may be having a toxic effect on you.

CHEMICAL POLLUTANTS OUTSIDE THE HOME

The worst chemical pollutants outside the home for someone with MS are diesel fumes and lead from gas exhaust fumes. Therefore, living in cities or near traffic-clogged arterial routes may be worse for you than living in a place with relatively clean air, such as the seaside.

These pollutants can also affect food on sale in produce shops situated on main roads near traffic lights. If the fruit and vegetables are displayed outside on the pavement in such a position, they are bound to be contaminated with the toxins given off by the traffic. The best thing is to avoid buying produce from such a shop.

ALTERNATIVES TO CHEMICALS

It is possible to find alternatives to all of the noxious chemicals mentioned.

Cleaning Agents

Choose an ecological brand that is biodegradable. Or use ordinary baking soda. Buy cans of polish instead of aerosols.

Toothpaste

Use bicarbonate of soda instead or a homeopathic brand.

Cosmetics and Toiletries

Use soap without coloring or scent. Use aloe vera shampoo and other cosmetics. Make sure that there are no detergents and no additives.

Water

Buy a water filter that can be connected to your water supply pipe and becomes like a "third tap" in your kitchen. This filters out all harmful substances in the drinking water supply. Or buy pure bottled spring water.

Furniture and Furnishings

Avoid chipboard. Avoid foam. Avoid synthetic fabrics. Go instead for solid wood and natural fibers in cushions and mattresses and also in fabrics for furnishings.

Bedding

As you spend about eight hours out of every twenty-four in bed, it is important for the bed to be uncontaminated by chemical pollutants. Ideally, the frame should be metal or hardwood.

Even a wood like pine gives off fumes, called terpenes. Be careful about the headboard, and avoid anything with foam or chipboard. Try to get a mattress made with natural fibers. If you have a foam mattress, cover it with old-fashioned cotton ticking. Go for pure cotton sheets, pillow cases, and duvet covers. Avoid polyester, which is a synthetic and part of the plastics family.

Gas Appliances

Ideally, site the hot water heater in an outhouse; otherwise, house it in a casing that will stop the fumes from getting into the kitchen. If necessary, improve the ventilation.

Clothes

Avoid synthetic fabrics and wool, which is often treated chemically. The best fabric is pure cotton. Avoid sending your clothes to the dry cleaners, as dry cleaning fluid gives off fumes. If you have to dry clean certain garments, air them thoroughly outdoors before wearing them. You could probably safely ignore some labels inside garments and wash them even though the label may say "dry clean only."

Where to Find Alternatives

Organic produce retailers often also supply other products, such as a range of biodegradable cleaning agents. Your local health food shop will probably have nonchemical cosmetics and toiletries, and so will some pharmacies.

OTHER POSSIBLE ENVIRONMENTAL POLLUTANTS

Of course, it is not just chemicals that can cause allergies. Troublesome particles in the air can be biological as well as chemical. The most common allergens in this category are:

- dust
- house dust mites

- mold spores
- pollens
- cat and dog dander

It is important to keep rooms clean and dusted, especially the bedroom.

ECOLOGY IN EVERYDAY LIFE

Apart from avoiding the chemicals listed, there are many other things you can do in your everyday life to make your environment healthier.

- Do not use aluminum saucepans or frying pans for cooking. If you have any, throw them out. Minute particles of aluminum can get into the food that you cook in these utensils. This has been associated with conditions such as senile dementia and Alzheimer's disease.
- Eat nothing out of cans. Metal particles can seep into the foods and contaminate them. It is always better to eat fresh foods anyway, with frozen as a second best.

The Contraceptive Pill

Dr. Ellen Grant, author of *The Bitter Pill* (Corgi, 1986) believes that the increasing incidence of MS, especially among young women, can be linked with the pill, which has been in widespread use since the mid-1960s. The pill, among its many other actions, robs the body of zinc. Any women with MS would be better off using a form of contraception that does not involve chemicals.

Microwaves from Transmitters

This theory comes from Sheffield scientist Dr. Jane G. Clarke, who has written a book called *Multiple Sclerosis—A New Theory Concerning Cause and Cure* (New Age Science Press, 1983). Her main thesis is that the damage seen in MS is due to overheating of the myelin sheath. The overheating is brought on by various factors, the most controversial one being microwaves, particularly radar waves in the 10-cm waveband, which bypass the skin's heat receptors. Dr. Clarke suggests that people who get MS have been brought up on a copper-deficient diet, so that their myelin never reaches normal thickness. More information can be obtained from

New Age Science Press Ltd.
66 Hatings Rd.
Millhouses
Sheffield S7 2GU, UK

Electrical Equipment

Theories about the effects of electrical equipment can be obtained from

Dr. Cyril Smith
Electrical Engineering Department
Salford University
Manchester, UK

Vaccinations

The view that vaccinations may be implicated in MS is shared by several holistic practitioners, including the late Dr. Robert S. Mendelsohn, editor of "The People's Doctor" (PO Box 982, Evanston, Illinois 60204). In volume 6, issue 5, of "The People's Doctor," Dr. Mendelsohn wrote:

> While scientists have spent millions of dollars in a fruitless chase of possible viruses that might cause MS, I believe the most overlooked area of research is that which doctors call iatrogenic (doctor-produced). Since it is highly unlikely that any miracle drug will be found, I would recommend that every MS researcher and all the various fund-raising organizations pursue factors that may prevent MS. High on my list of suspicious doctor-caused factors are delayed reactions to infant formula, routine immunizations, and allergy shots. After all, we now know that another serious neurologic

condition, Guillain-Barré paralysis, comes from the swine flu vaccine and other vaccines.

Another alternative practitioner who shares this view is Leon Chaitow, whose book *Vaccination and Immunisation: Dangers, Delusions and Alternatives* (C.W. Daniel) was nominated as a book of the year by the *Journal of Alternative Medicine* in the UK.

Many people with MS report that their first symptoms followed shortly after some vaccination, such as smallpox. This may or may not be coincidental.

It is probably safer to avoid any further vaccinations once MS is diagnosed, even though this might restrict visiting certain countries. If you can stand your ground against doctors, you might also consider saying no to all vaccinations for your children (except those for tetanus and polio).

13

Hyperbaric Oxygen Treatment

WHAT IS HYPERBARIC OXYGEN?

Hyperbaric oxygen (HBO) is oxygen at an increased level of pressure. "Hyper" means increased; "baric" means pressure. You go into a special chamber with increased atmospheric pressure and breathe oxygen through a mask. Under increased pressure, there is a higher concentration of oxygen coming in contact with and saturating tissue and blood. All cells of the body are bathed in this oxygen.

The special chambers used for hyperbaric oxygen treatment look like big metal capsules. A typical one has six or eight seats with portholes. Each seat is equipped with an oxygen feed to which an oxygen mask is connected. During the treatment (sometimes called a "dive"), you put this oxygen mask over your mouth and nose and breathe pure oxygen.

How Does It Work?

No one knows for sure. One of the most popular theories is that of Dr. Philip James of Dundee University. He is a consultant in occupational medicine who specializes in diving. He says that MS may result from fatty blockages in tiny blood vessels. The medical term for this is "fat globule micro-embolism."

Dr. James believes that fat embolism, blockage by fat globules, is responsible for the damage to blood vessels at the onset of every new MS symptom. The damaged vessels leak toxic substances into the surrounding nerve tissues, damaging the myelin sheaths and producing the scattered scars of multiple sclerosis in the central nervous system. If Dr. James's fatty blockage theory is right, HBO treatment works because oxygen, when breathed under pressure, dislodges the fat globules and disperses them.

Interestingly, divers who get "the bends" when they come up from a deep sea dive too fast suffer from symptoms very similar to MS. Their symptoms are the result of air bubbles in the circulation. Dr. James suggests that fat globules in the blood block blood vessels in the nervous system in the same way in multiple sclerosis. However, this theory may be only part of the story.

When Dr. Richard Neubauer, a doctor practicing hyperbaric oxygen medicine in Florida, gave a talk on HBO to ARMS in 1983, he listed several possible different ways HBO might be working (Figure 11). He was certain that the oxygen gets right to the nucleus of cells. In addition, it regenerates nerve axons, it has good effects on the body's immune system, it reduces or stops swelling in the central nervous system, it increases microcirculation, and it even improves IQ.

Of course, oxygen is vital for healthy people too. It is necessary for all body tissues, but especially sensitive nerve tissue. If the oxygen level in the blood of a healthy person drops, the blood vessels in the brain dilate and eventually leak, causing brain swelling due to the build-up of liquid.

In the USA, hyperbaric oxygen is commonly used in the treatment of about forty conditions. This long list includes drowning, diving accidents, burns, crash injuries, severed limbs, electrocution, smoke inhalation, and cyanide poisoning.

HBO treatment doesn't produce major changes overnight. Increased oxygenation simply allows the natural mechanisms of repair in the body to take place.

What's the Treatment Like?

Of course, what it feels like to have HBO treatment does differ somewhat from person to person. Even so, there are some broad guidelines.

FIGURE 11
How HBO May Be Working

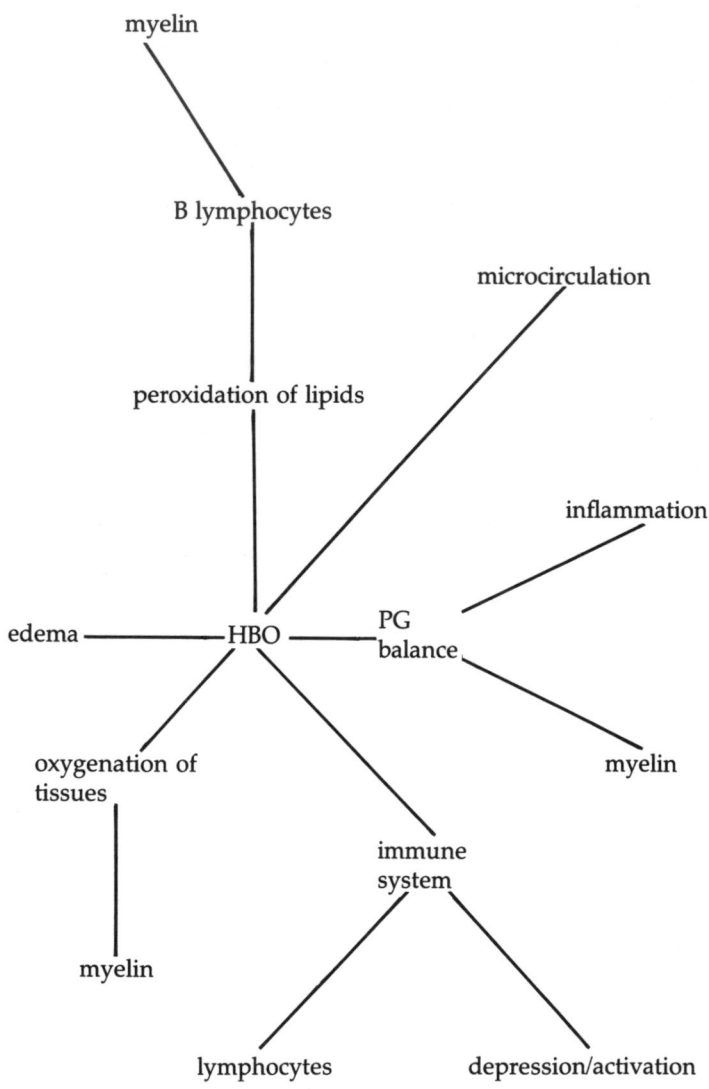

You are seated in the chamber with other people having the treatment. When everyone is settled, the chamber operators begin the "descent." They tell you when to put on your mask and begin breathing oxygen. Most chambers have an intercom system so that the operators can keep you informed about what is happening and you can tell them if there are any problems.

Gradually, the operators increase the pressure inside the chamber. This process can take up to ten minutes, and it's the only part of the treatment that can be a little bit unpleasant. It's rather like going deep underground in a subway or taking off in an airplane—your ears pop. The trick is to keep swallowing.

Once you're "down" (you don't go anywhere—it's just that the atmosphere has changed so that it's like being deep under the sea), you stay for about an hour and a half. All you do is sit there, with your mask on, breathing oxygen. Many people like to take along books or magazines to help pass the time.

In some treatment centers, there is a "half-time" during which you can take off your mask, have a bit of a rest, and breathe normal air. By the way, the air in the chamber at all times feels perfectly normal both to sit in and to breathe, despite the change in atmospheric pressure.

At the end of the treatment period, the operators slowly bring you "up" to sea level—again taking about ten minutes. Once the pressure inside the chamber is the same as the air outside, the air-locked door can be opened and out you go.

How Many Treatments Do You Need? And at What Depth?

How many treatments you should have, how deep you should go, and exactly how much oxygen you should breathe have not been standardized. It seems that what works for one person may not be ideal for another, so that, with the help of the chamber operators who will be monitoring you, you may have to find the best method for you.

When HBO treatments first started, it was thought that the depth should be thirty-three feet, which is known as "two atmospheres." The best course of treatments was thought to be twenty-one dives, one each day, taken on consecutive days, six days a week.

Over the last couple of years, however, there has been experimentation with depths and lengths of treatment, so that now you are likely to be able to choose the depth that works best for you and go into the chamber with people of similar need.

Now dives can be eight, ten, sixteen, twenty-four, or thirty-three feet. Some treatments can be over a period of three weeks; others over five weeks. A dose of oxygen can be altered by adjusting the pressure of air in the chamber or by adjusting the amount of oxygen coming into the mask.

Why Do You Have to Be in a Chamber at All?

People often ask why you can't just breathe oxygen sitting at home in an armchair. The answer is that, when you breathe oxygen at normal pressures, you cannot reach the same oxygen content in the blood as when you breathe oxygen under increased pressure. Using oxygen at an increased atmospheric pressure reduces the diameter of blood vessels in the nervous system. Despite the reduction in blood flow, the delivery of oxygen to the tissues is in fact increased. This may sound like a paradox, but it's true.

Top-Ups

From the research done thus far, it seems that "top-ups," or maintenance treatments, are essential to any improvement and keep the disease stable. How often you have a top-up does vary from person to person. For some people, it could be as often as twice a week, particularly for those people with fluctuating symptoms. For others, whose conditions are more stable, it could be every ten days or longer. The pressure level in the top-up sessions is usually the same as that used in the initial treatment course.

Dr. James says that HBO should be thought of as a supplement, a bit like insulin to a diabetic. So top-up treatments should not be neglected, in case old symptoms come back.

Hints during HBO Treatment

- Eat a nutritious diet (see Chapter 3). Have something to eat and drink before you go into the chamber.
- It can be colder inside the chamber than in the outer room, so wear comfortable, warm clothes, but don't wear any nylon or other static-prone materials that might create a spark. Take off your watch, as the increased pressure inside the chamber can cause the cover of the watch face to pop off.
- Give a list of all drugs and medications that you are taking to the operators.
- Tell them if you have a bad cold, as this can make the ear problems worse. You might be advised to skip a treatment or two until the cold is gone.
- There are divided views on whether you should be allowed to have sweets or gum, as you might when a plane is taking off or landing. Many people have found that swallowing does lessen the ear problems, but some centers have found that moving the jaw has interfered with the oxygen masks. So you had better ask your operators about this.
- Take a good book, magazines, crossword puzzles, or whatever will keep you from getting bored. The lighting is bright enough to read.
- Cigarette smoking is absolutely forbidden either in the chamber or in the centers. Nothing flammable may be taken inside the chamber and no petroleum-based products may be worn on the body.

DOES HBO WORK?

No one is claiming that HBO is a cure for MS. To be realistic, HBO can't instantly put to right long-term deterioration. Many people do respond once the right pressure and the right length of treatment have been found. It seems that even the patients who don't improve can sometimes remain stable. If it achieves nothing else, HBO may be able to stabilize MS.

However, there is no doubt that some people do improve as

a result of HBO. Dr. Richard Neubauer says, "The changes are so obvious, an idiot could see them." Unfortunately, these changes don't happen to everyone.

The most positive research thus far comes from Dr. Boguslav Fischer and his colleagues at the New York University Medical Center. The study was published in the *New England Journal of Medicine* in 1982. In the group who were given HBO, there was an immediate improvement in twelve of seventeen. In the control group, there was an improvement in only one of twenty. After a year, deterioriation was noticed in two patients in the HBO group and eleven patients in the control group. The good results from the HBO treatment wore off in seven of the treated group but were long-lasting in five.

Dr. Fischer himself is quoted as saying the HBO produces "a possible slowing of the progression of the disease." He concluded, however, that more research is needed. "This therapy cannot be generally recommended without longer follow-up periods and additional confirmatory experience."

A leading place for HBO in the UK is Dundee, largely because Dr. Philip James is at Dundee University and also because ARMS has a particularly active HBO center there, which was the first in the UK.

In 1983, a pilot study was conducted by Dr. Duncan Davison of Dundee for ARMS, although this was not a controlled trial. The results were not wonderful, but not bad. Of thirty-eight patients (eleven male, twenty-seven female), a third reported improvements in bladder function, sensation, and muscle coordination during the three weeks after HBO treatment. These people did not improve in other MS symptoms.

Thirteen patients described feeling better during treatment, and this improvement started at any time between the first treatment and the seventeenth treatment. One patient described herself as feeling mentally hyperactive for several hours after each session.

On the Disability Status Scale (a measure for physical disability), four patients improved by 1 point and were considered to be moderately improved. Some patients noted differences in their motor function that made a significant difference in their daily life. Four patients described an important increase in the distance they could walk before they got fatigued. For example, a person who used to be able to walk only three hundred yards before HBO treatment could walk a mile after it. In two of these patients, however, there was deterioration within seven days of the end of the treatment. In one, the deterioration was so significant that he was worse than before the treatment started. These are some of the remarks made by the patients who noticed improvement in their motor functions, such as walking and moving their arms: "less trailing of the legs when walking," "less footdrop in the right leg," "increased power in the hand," "slight increase in power," "writing better."

A third of the patients noted an improvement in what neurologists call "cerebellar function"—nodding of the head, shakiness, unsteadiness. The improvements were less shakiness and the ability to stand on a chair or to stand up without feeling unsteady. No patient had a dramatic improvement in "cerebellar function," and two got worse.

Fourteen patients had improved sensory functions—44 percent of the total. These people noted loss of the "bandaged" feeling under the chest, return of feeling to hands or fingers, and lessening of pain in the limbs. On the other hand, five patients went the other way and suffered loss of sensation, more pain, more tingling, and more numbness. As compared to the 44 percent who improved, 3 percent worsened.

In bowel and bladder functions, there was improvement in ten patients, or 37 percent. No patient got worse in bladder function. There was no significant change in bowel function. In the group in which bladder function improved, one patient said that he used to have to go to the toilet every hour before the HBO, but only needed to go once every four to five hours after the HBO. Another said that she used to have to get up two or three times in the night and now she had to get up only once or not at all. Another said that her visits to the toilet had reduced from once every one to one and a half hours to once every two or three hours, with less urgency. There is no doubt from the

Davison study that the clearest benefits were in bladder symptoms.

Dr. Davison's conclusion follows.

> Improvement in approximatively one third of patients with bladder symptoms, sensory symptoms and ataxia were described, but no benefit overall in other functions. The changes appear to be greater than may be anticipated from the placebo response, suggesting that hyperbaric oxygen does have an effect on the nervous system.

However, striking results were reported by Dr. Neubauer in the USA. In one study (1980) of two hundred fifty patients with MS, he reported a "dramatic" improvement in 39 percent, minimal and moderate improvement in 52 percent, and no improvement in 9 percent. He reported similar results in another study (1982) of six hundred patients, where the experience of his own unit was pooled with patients being treated in Houston, Texas, and Naples, Italy.

Recent Research on HBO

Research during the period 1982–1986 has not been able to repeat the good results of Fischer and Neubauer in the USA. Indeed, recent research trials on HBO have found there is no significant benefit *overall* in MS with HBO treatment.

Two major trials in the UK were commissioned by the MS Society of Great Britain and N. Ireland, one in Newcastle and the other at St. Thomas's Hospital and Whipps Cross Hospital in London. The Newcastle results were published in the *Lancet* in February 1985; the London results were published in the *British Medical Journal* in February 1986. Both trials could find no significant benefit of HBO on overall MS symptoms. However, the Newcastle trial did find a small but significant subjective improvement in bladder function.

The London study of eighty-four patients could find no clinically important or significant benefit in the patient's subjective opinion, the examiner's opinion, the score on the Kurtzke disability status scale, or the time taken to walk 50 meters. All of the doctors involved in these major trials reached the same conclusion—that HBO is not an effective treatment for MS. The authors of the paper published in the *British Medical Journal* concluded that

> The results . . . on a total of 204 patients studied under double blind conditions in the United Kingdom fit in with the findings of several smaller studies recently reported in the USA . . . our findings, obtained with detailed methods of assessment . . . have failed to confirm those of Fischer *et al.* There appears to be little basis for recommending this treatment to patients with multiple sclerosis.

David Bates, Professor of Neurology at the Royal Victoria Infirmary in Newcastle, was one of the doctors on the Newcastle study. He feels that the negative result from these two major studies should refute once and for all the suggestion that HBO should be part of the management of MS.

Despite these trials, the controversy still continues. Those who support HBO still do so, challenging those doctors who feel that they have proved it ineffective.

One of the main supporters of HBO is Dr. Philip James of Dundee. He criticizes the Newcastle and London trials on various scores. First, the patients were treated at 2 atmospheres absolute, which may be too much; second, the patients in the trials were not given top-ups, which he considers very important; third, he thinks that the patients selected for the trials should not have been chronic cases. He argues that HBO may be best suited for *acute* cases of MS.

The other therapeutic uses for HBO are in acute circumstances. Dr. James feels that it is indefensible to wait for a patient to get worse—to the point where the condition is irreversible—before starting treatment. As with all therapies, Dr. James claims that HBO works best for those patients who are not yet badly disabled. In answer to Dr. James's criticisms, the doctors involved in the two large UK trials say that they followed very closely the protocol of the Fischer study in the USA, which had such favorable results.

The poor results of HBO for MS as reported from Newcastle

and London do not tally with other results, particularly from Italy. Professor Damiano Zannini and others from the Hyperbaric Medicine Center in Genoa, Italy, found that HBO is beneficial for MS patients. They concluded that

- improvements or regression of symptoms, or functional recovery, can be observed;
- these improvements can be lasting or temporary;
- a trend toward the disease worsening was halted;
- the symptoms most likely to improve were cerebellar (e.g., shakiness, unsteadiness, head nodding), sensory, and sphincteric (bladder and bowel control).

Professor Zannini did feel that HBO is still an experimental treatment, until further research is done.

Bladder and Bowel Control

What seems to be emerging from various trials is that the symptoms most helped by HBO are bladder and bowel control. Even the Bates trial in Newcastle, which found no *overall* benefit of HBO, did find that it helped bladder and bowel symptoms. Twelve of fifty-one patients in the HBO group, compared with only three of the forty-seven control patients, felt that the HBO had helped their bladder and bowel symptoms.

Other studies done in various parts of the world back up these results—25 to 50 percent of patients on HBO report improvement in bladder and bowel function. Dr. Appell in Louisiana and Dr. Neubauer in Florida draw particular attention to improvements in bladder and bowel function.

This improvement in bladder function was somewhat glossed over by the Newcastle doctors in their report in the *Lancet*. This is challenged by Dr. Philip James:

Objective evidence of improvement in bladder function with hyperbaric oxygen therapy has been produced by urologists under double-blind conditions. It is clearly wrong to discount the importance of bladder function in the management of patients with chronic multiple sclerosis, in view of the associated morbidity and the effects of bladder dysfunction on the quality of life.

"Subjective" Results—The ARMS Study

Normally, patients in medical trials are assessed objectively by specialists, and "subjective" assessments tend not to be taken into consideration (although they were considered in the trial done at St. Thomas's and Whipps Cross Hospitals). ARMS decided to look at HBO from the patients' subjective point of view, i.e., how they themselves felt about the treatment. Fifty participants filled in questionnaires that covered much wider aspects of health than is usually covered. The questions included areas of personal and social life, as well as physical and psychological health.

The participants in this trial were divided into two groups, A and B. Each group had an eight-week regimen of HBO plus top-ups (regime 1) and then crossed over to an eight-week regimen of air plus top-ups (regime 2). This is called a double-blind, controlled, crossover trial. In all, the participants had twenty treatments of HBO plus top-ups and sixteen treatments of air.

Although there was little evidence of improvement related specifically to HBO, most participants did report effects that they themselves attributed to HBO. Participants from different social backgrounds responded differently to the trial. There were significant changes for the better reported in relation to sleeping better, having more energy, feeling less socially isolated, and having a more rewarding social life. On specific MS symptoms, the majority felt that they had improved. Increased mobility and improved urinary symptoms were the two areas that people said had improved most.

There is a very big difference between the HBO therapy given at ARMS centers around England and the HBO treatment given as part of the Newcastle and London trials. Going to the HBO chamber in an ARMS center is a social event. You meet people and make friends. You share the experience in a multi-chamber with several other people. The chamber becomes a friendly place, a place where people can tell jokes, play card games, chat, or just read.

In the big trials, the HBO was just a treatment. Indeed, at St. Thomas's and Whipps Cross Hospitals, the HBO was in single, one-person chambers, so there was no chance of any sociability attached to the therapy. Perhaps one of the therapeutic aspects of the kind of HBO given at ARMS centers is that it is like a club; people's spirits are raised and they feel better—both mentally and physically.

ARMS HBO Centers—Anecdotal Reports

The results of recent scientific trials into HBO have not been good, but you could visit any ARMS HBO center anywhere in the country and hear stories of people making dramatic improvements. There are anecdotes of people who went into the chamber in a wheelchair and came out walking. On the other hand, you would also hear stories of people gaining no improvement whatsover.

Most stories would relate minor improvements, such as being able to hold a cup without shaking or gaining longer intervals between visits to the toilet. This sort of mild improvement in activities of daily living would not feature in the results of a big scientific trial, where one needs to move up a point on the Disability Scale before improvements are considered significant, yet for someone to be able to hold a cup without spilling its content *is* a major improvement in their daily quality of life.

No one is claiming that HBO is a cure for MS. Despite the trial results, however, it may help to stabilize or improve some symptoms of MS. The less disabled you are, the greater the chance of HBO being of benefit.

Neurological Benefits in the ARMS Trial

Dr. Alec Forti, the neurologist at the ARMS Unit at the Central Middlesex Hospital, made some interesting analyses from the

ARMS trial. He concluded that there were no large benefits from HBO if you took the groups studied as a whole. Once you broke down the big groups into subgroups, however, there were some benefits. The most significant improvements were in eye-hand coordination and peak flow.

SHOULD HBO BE GIVEN TO EARLY CASES AND ACUTE CASES OF MS?

Again, if the results of trials are analyzed in a different way, the picture that emerges is that the recently diagnosed and those with a slower course of the disease without any irreversible disability show the highest percentage of improvement from HBO therapy. Professor Pallotta, from Naples, Italy, followed one hundred MS patients on HBO therapy between 1977 and 1981. He concluded that "the clinical case with a slower course and those recently diagnosed showed the highest percentage of improvement."

Dr. Philip James, in a letter sent to the *British Medical Journal* in February 1986, argued very strongly for early treatment with HBO. He is very angry that only chronically disabled patients were selected for the big trials on HBO. He wrote: "The wisdom in choosing chronically disabled patients in trials of therapy in multiple sclerosis, or indeed for trials of therapy in any disease, must be challenged."

Dr. James said that symptoms present for a short time are much more likely to remit given oxygen therapy than are long-term problems. Rather than wait for a patient to be incurably scarred before even making a diagnosis, Dr. James urges that doctors refer patients for HBO therapy as soon as someone suffers an acute attack. He feels that if patients suffering acute attacks were given immediate HBO, there would be hope of preventing further disability. However, people with MS who had recently suffered an acute attack were excluded from the big trials.

Dr. James is very critical of those in the medical establishment who sit back and allow an acute condition to turn into a chronic condition. He says: "We need to remove the ridiculous and self-defeating requirement for multiple lesions to be present before trials of therapy can be undertaken."

IS HBO SAFE?

In all the fuss in Britain about HBO, there have been some press reports suggesting that people with MS could be "burnt alive" in pressurized oxygen chambers. This is nonsense. It is true that certain hyperbaric oxygen chambers used in hospitals don't use oxygen masks but fill the whole chamber with oxygen. In this situation, a spark could ignite with disastrous results. The HBO chambers as used by local ARMS groups are not like that. The chambers are filled with ordinary room air. The only pure oxygen is from the masks, and basic precautions are taken to eliminate any possibility of a spark. In addition, both the UK and the US governments inspect pressure vessels and approve them for human occupancy.

The other issue over which there is some controversy is whether there should be professional technicians operating the chambers. In fact, the chambers are quite easy to operate. The ARMS centers in the UK have many volunteers, most of whom are family or friends of someone with MS. As operators of the chambers they are especially involved, concerned, and caring people.

However, some experts feel that it is essential to have trained technicians operating the chambers. In the US, an accredited course is currently being developed to train qualified HBO operators. US authorities also stress that treatments should be taken on the recommendation and under the jurisdiction of a physician.

Does HBO Have Side Effects?

Probably the most common side effect is ear-popping (Table 3). In some people, this can be worse than the sensation you get in your ears when a plane takes off or lands. This side effect is lessened if the operator alters the pressure in the chamber very slowly going down and coming up again. The operators normally hold the chamber at a certain pressure level for a little while before going on to the next. This allows the people inside the chamber to get used to each pressure level.

The other common side effect is on the eyes. The oxygen affects the lens of the eye so that for a short time you may not be able to see as well as normal. This side effect usually disappears within an hour or so after each treatment.

Sleepiness is another frequently mentioned side effect. However, this sleepiness often indicates that improvement is taking place. This terrible tiredness tends to affect different people at different stages of the treatment. For some, it can happen during the first week; for others, during the last week.

Because tiredness is so common for the first week or so of the treatment, it's important to plan absolutely nothing that could tire you during the HBO course. It would also be sensible to ask someone to drive you home because your vision may not be up to it for an hour or so after the treatment.

However, once the tiredness phase has passed, people frequently report a feeling of extra energy and liveliness. Some people experience the "high" of oxygen, in which you feel elated or euphoric. Unfortunately, this pleasant side effect doesn't last.

TABLE 3
Unwanted Effects of HBO, St. Thomas's Hospital and Whipps Cross Hospital Trials

A total of 84 patients took part in the trials.

	HBO Group	Placebo Group
Ear discomfort	26 (3 severe)	10
Deafness	8	3
Sinus pain	2	1
Headache	4	4
Leg Pain	5	4
Visual disturbance	8	3
Nausea	3	1
Fatigue	16	20
Fear or anxiety	9 (2 severe)	5

Another thing that can happen is that, when you do get sensations back, ironically, they might actually feel bad. For example, when an area of numb skin regains its sensation, you may feel "pins and needles."

In the Dundee study, apart from the ear problems, two patients said that they had a bigger appetite; one lost appetite and thirteen pounds in weight. Two patients complained of vertigo and light-headedness as a result of HBO. One patient developed migraine attacks during some treatments. Fatigue was said to increase in nine patients and decrease in nine patients.

The London study, reported in February 1986 in the *British Medical Journal*, found that unwanted side effects were quite common in both the group given HBO and the group given just air. Minor ear discomfort was the commonest problem, but no patient had long-lasting side effects to their ears. Visual disturbances consisted of blurring of vision, usually toward the end of the treatment, which lasted thirty minutes to six hours after treatment, but for several days in one case. One patient remarked on a disturbance of color vision after HBO treatment. Two patients became anxious and claustrophobic and had to withdraw from treatment. After ear problems, fatigue was the most common side effect.

Anti-oxidants

Some doctors think that it is important to take anti-oxidants—vitamins E and C in particular—when undergoing HBO treatment. This lessens the risk of free radicals (see page 78).

HBO CENTERS

Lee Palmer
Hyperbaric Oxygen Therapy
Service
212 South Wilson Avenue
Barstow, FL 33830
813-533-4862

Jane Dunne
Hyperbark Oxygen Unit
Undersea Medical Society
9650 Rockville Pike
Bethesda, MD 20814
301-530-9226

14

Physical Therapy and Exercise

Many people with MS are more disabled than they need to be. It is *not* part of the disease process of MS to have backs bent forward, arms or legs stuck in unnatural positions (contractures), or atrophied leg mucles. These things develop only because of repeated misuse and inactivity.

One of the many scandals with MS is that doctors do not refer their patients to physical therapists early enough or in anything but an *ad hoc* way. Nor do they usually suggest that activity is much better than inactivity. Even if a doctor does diagnose MS, he is much more likely to say "Just go away and forget about it" than to say that physical therapy and exercise can help.

Patients with MS who are referred to physical therapists are usually referred too late. It is much easier to maintain existing use of limbs than to regain the use of limbs that have become disabled.

Once again, it is a case of shutting the stable door after the horse has bolted. How much saner it would be if people with MS could receive all possible treatments very early in the disease, before permanent damage has been done.

Studies have now proved that certain treatments *are* effective and should be started as early in the disease as possible. Physical therapy/exercise is one of the therapies that has been shown to have real benefit.

WHY PHYSICAL THERAPY/EXERCISE IS SO IMPORTANT

- It improves circulation and all bodily functions.
- It increases the amount of oxygen in the blood.
- It keeps muscles strong and strengthens weak ones.
- It keeps joints mobile and prevents stiffness.
- It may help reduce spasticity.
- It helps maintain maximal independence.
- It lifts depression.
- It gives a feeling of well-being by toning up the whole system.
- It prevents muscles from atrophying.
- It helps you do everyday things better.
- It gives you more energy.
- It helps you look good.
- It helps keep at bay disabilities that are not part of the MS disease process.

If You Don't Use It, You Lose It

Our motto should be "If you don't use it, you lose it." Another good one is "Make the best of what you've got."

Many of the complications of MS arise from disuse. Contractures, deformities, and reduced mobility are often simply put down to being part of having MS, but they are not necessarily part of the disease process at all. They come about because of misuse and disuse.

Inactivity can lead to complications. On the other hand, activity can prevent complications or at least delay them.

Regular exercising can make the difference between being able to stand and to walk—or becoming wheelchair-bound.

Fatigue

You may think that you haven't got the energy to do any sort of exercise and fear that it would make you feel drained. The ironic thing about exercise, however, is that it energizes you. Of course, you shouldn't exert yourself so much that you're exhausted, but no exercise at all will leave you more fatigued than gentle exercise, which keeps the body in good tone.

Exercises are designed not only to increase fitness, but also to increase stamina and endurance. Stamina will take time to build up but will make you fatigue less easily.

You will learn your own limits of endurance. Stop before you get fatigued, or there could be detrimental effects. Keep cool while exercising to stave off fatigue caused by heat.

Any gross lack of regular exercise causes disuse atrophy. Research has shown that muscle disuse due to immobility results in the selective atrophy of the slow, oxidative, fatigue-resistant type I muscle fiber, as opposed to the fast-fatiguing, glucolytic type II fibers.

However, regular exercise changes the biochemical properties of skeletal muscles. Endurance training in particular partially converts the type II fibers from anaerobic to aerobic metabolism, making them more fatigue-resistant—or more like type I fibers.

EXERCISE YOU CAN DO ON YOUR OWN

If you are active enough to do exercises on your own, you may not need to see a physical therapist. You can do on your own whatever exercise you enjoy doing most. Possibilities are

- walking
- swimming
- dancing
- exercise classes, including stretching and gentle aerobics
- rebounder exercises

A rebounder, which looks like a minitrampoline, is very good for building up strength in your leg muscles and for stamina. If you have a problem with balance, you can put the rebounder near a wall so you can touch the wall to keep your balance. You will be amazed at how quickly your jumping ability increases, just by using the rebounder for a couple of minutes every day.

Whatever exercise you choose, do it regularly, ideally every day. It will make a real, noticeable difference to your strength and stamina.

Always stop exercising before you get tired. Never allow yourself to get fatigued.

WHY YOU SHOULD SEE A PHYSICAL THERAPIST EARLY ON

If you see a physical therapist early on, she or he will be able to prevent secondary handicap—the sort of handicap that is not part of MS but is a preventable complication of it. The therapist will help you keep your present abilities or even improve on them.

A physical therapist will design a tailor-made set of exercises just for you, which you can then do on your own, ideally every day. Ideally, a physical therapist or therapists should continue their involvement with you, taking into account the fluctuations of the disease. At present, patients are rarely referred to a physical therapist at all, or perhaps only as part of a stay in the hospital. If no one suggests it, ask your doctor to refer you to a physical therapist at your local hospital.

If your particular problems could be identified early on, the physical therapist could work with you on those problems and stop them from developing into something worse. The aim would be to work out a program so that you could maintain or improve your present abilities—all of your movements and all your activities of daily living. Physical therapists talk about "maintaining a level of function."

A Partnership between Patient and Physical Therapist

In a good partnership between a patient and a physical therapist, the patient is not just passively on the receiving end of treatment but is actively involved and responsible. This means seeing the management of multiple sclerosis as a way of life, rather than just a series of therapies. It also means understanding the benefits of rest, as well as the benefits of activity. It means not being lazy and doing the exercises designed for you.

A physical therapist will teach you how to stand properly, how to balance properly, how to stand up from sitting and lying, how to walk properly, how to position yourself to sleep, and how to coordinate your movements better. He or she will help you be aware of your posture, your movements, and your sensory perception.

There is a right way and a wrong way of doing all of these things, and a physical therapist will teach you the right way to avoid bad habits. The aim is to bring your body back into balance so you can move more normally and freely and enjoy an active life as long as possible.

POSTURE, SECONDARY HANDICAP, AND EXERCISE

A poor posture may be the first sign of muscle imbalance (Figures 12 to 14). It may be hard to stand up properly because of damage to neural mechanisms. It is very important to take steps to correct bad posture because it can have a domino effect: apart from throwing the body out of balance, it also has a bad effect on breathing and on the internal organs, which will make constipation and incontinence worse than need be. A slouched posture also can cause pains in the neck and shoulders, depression, and flabby muscles. In time, postural abnormalities will have an effect on movement. All of these are examples of secondary handicap, which can be avoided.

The best way to prevent postural abnormalities from becoming fixed is a regular, daily stretching routine. A physical therapist will give you some simple stretching exercises to do every day at home. These stretching exercises will stimulate good posture and good balance. Yoga is also very good for correcting postural faults (see Chapter 15).

Balance

The loss of balance typical of MS may be due to abnormalities in the inner ear caused by the disease itself. However, walking as if you're falling off a tightrope could also be because of very bad posture. You are literally thrown off balance because your

FIGURE 12
Poor Posture

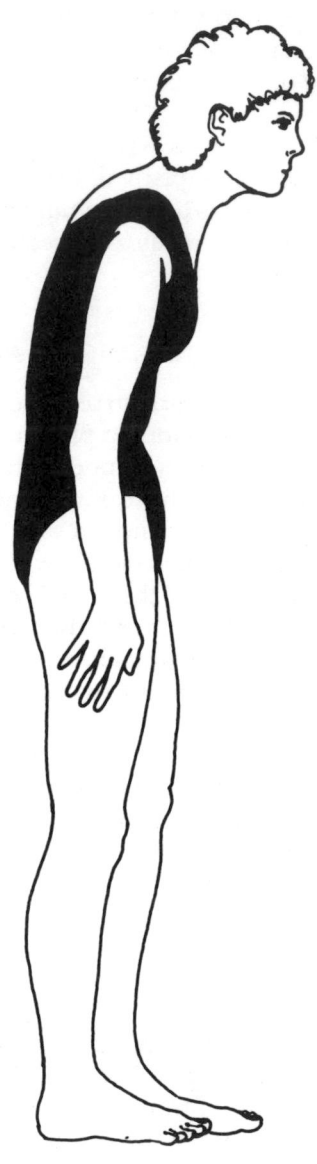

FIGURE 13
Good Posture

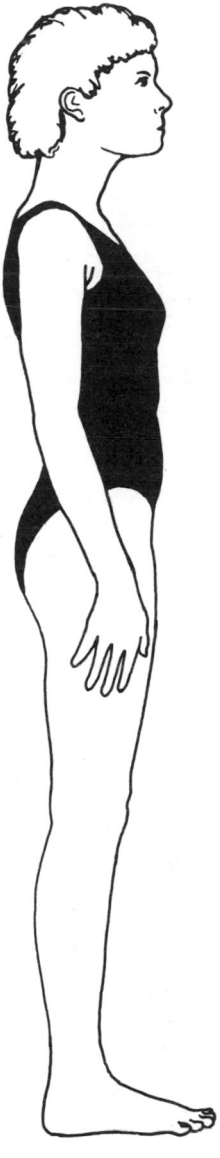

FIGURE 14
Good and Bad Posture in a Wheelchair

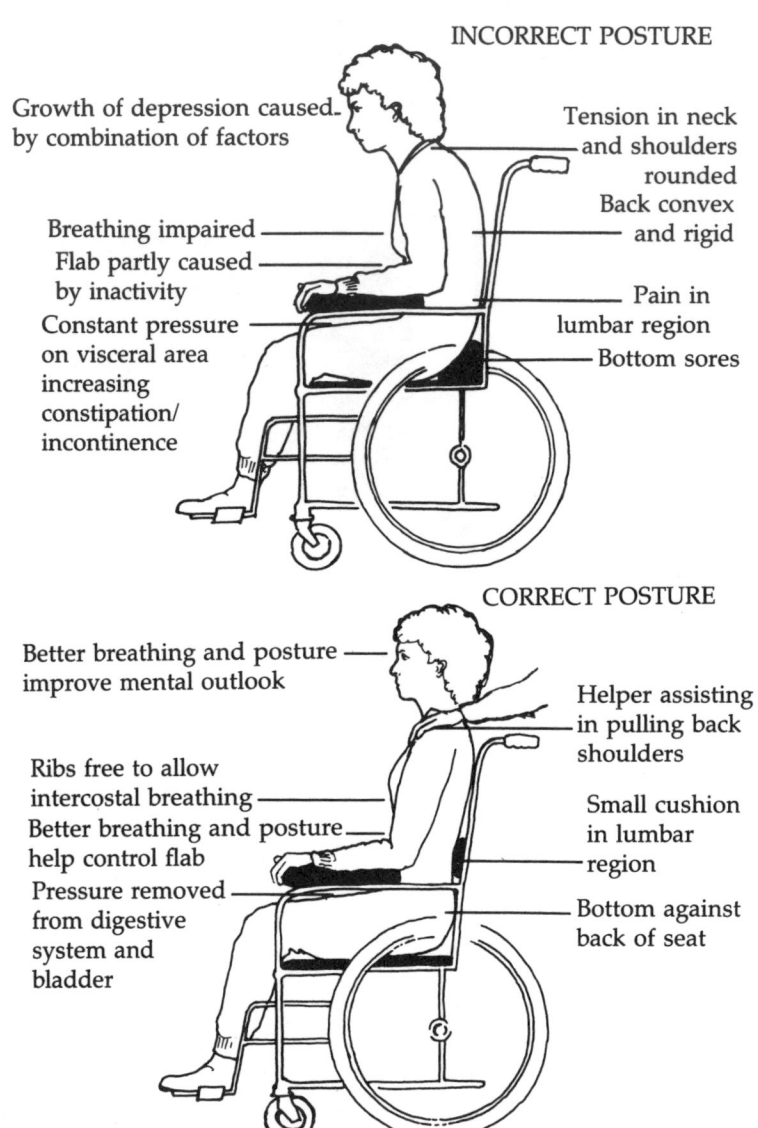

INCORRECT POSTURE

Growth of depression caused by combination of factors

Tension in neck and shoulders rounded

Back convex and rigid

Breathing impaired

Flab partly caused by inactivity

Constant pressure on visceral area increasing constipation/ incontinence

Pain in lumbar region

Bottom sores

CORRECT POSTURE

Better breathing and posture improve mental outlook

Helper assisting in pulling back shoulders

Ribs free to allow intercostal breathing

Better breathing and posture help control flab

Small cushion in lumbar region

Pressure removed from digestive system and bladder

Bottom against back of seat

body is out of alignment, and the center of gravity simply falls outside the base of support. To get yourself centered again, the physical therapist will suggest activities and exercises that stimulate balance. Yoga is also very good for this.

Muscle Tone

One of the things a physical therapist will identify is abnormalities in muscle tone, as they can create problems with movement. As with bad balance, poor muscle tone can be a secondary effect of poor posture. In people suffering from MS, muscles can be flaccid, with no tone, or the opposite, spastic, or else atrophied from disuse.

If the muscles have too much tone (i.e., are spastic), the physical therapist will design a program that avoids positions and activities that increase tone or reinforce abnormal ways of moving. The program will include daily walking or standing, carrying weights, and regular stretching. The therapist will also advise on how to avoid pressure sores, constipation, and bladder infections.

One of the things that is *not* helpful is to increase the strength of muscles that are strong already. This only makes the weaker ones weaker. If, for example, you are strong from the waist upward but weak from the waist downward, there is the temptation to use your arms and trunk a lot, not your legs and lower half.

There is a theory about "associated reactions" that goes like this: the more you use your right hand, the weaker your left hand gets; the more you use your arms, the weaker your legs get; one part of your body may well be compensating for another part. Concentrate on the weak areas; the strong areas can take care of themselves. That way you have the chance of bringing your body back into balance. If you only build up the strong muscles, the weak ones stand no chance, and the more out of balance you will be. That is why you should be careful not to put your weight on your hands when you sit down or get up from an armchair. Use your legs as much as you can.

WHAT EXERCISES?

A physical therapist will design a set of exercises tailor-made to your particular needs and disability. Gentle stretching exercises are likely to be part of this. Such exercises will be designed to make the most of what you've got, correct any postural faults, get you back on balance, and rectify abnormal muscle tone.

There is also nothing to stop you doing any kind of exercise that appeals to you. Obviously, what exercise you do depends on how disabled you are. Some people who have MS can play squash; others are grateful to be able to touch their toes while sitting in their wheelchair.

If you are able to move easily, there is no reason why you should not join an ordinary gym in your local area. Tell the instructor that you have MS so you will not be forced to do things beyond your ability or stamina and so that you can rest when you feel like it.

Any form of exercise will do you good. It does not have to be a formal class. If you have the self-discipline, you could exercise at home. Whatever you do, do it regularly. Ideally, every day.

Swimming is the best form of exercise and is ideal for disabled people as long as the water is hotter than in normal pools. Inquire whether there are any special swimming pools or swimming sessions in your area.

RESEARCH IN PHYSICAL THERAPY

The physical therapists at the ARMS Unit at the Central Middlesex Hospital conducted a retrospective study to find out whether physical therapy had any beneficial effects on the symptoms of MS. The results were very clear: the patients who had the most physical therapy—averaging eight hours per month—did best. The ones who had the least physical therapy—averaging half an hour a month—did the worst. The physical therapists did assessments of the patients in these areas: the voluntary control of a range of lower limb movements; activities such as getting in and out of bed, in and out of chairs, etc.; balance activities; and activities of daily living.

In all, forty patients took part in this study. All had been attending for physical therapy at the ARMS Unit for longer than a year. They all had a definite diagnosis of MS, none had suffered a relapse over a period of eighteen months, all of them had some problems with movement, and none of them suffered from any other condition that would have complicated the picture. The patients were assessed every six months over an eighteen-month period.

One of the observations of the physical therapists was that the patients' general condition got steadily worse, even though they did not suffer actual relapses. Changes in the group of forty showed that there was a highly significant progression toward greater disability with a loss of range in voluntary movements in the lower limbs.

On the other hand, the patients generally stayed the same in functional and also in balance activities. In activities of daily living, there were some real improvements toward more independence. The greatest changes were made in the first six months.

At one point the physical therapists changed the emphasis of the treatment to include more functional activities. At another point the emphasis was switched to balance activities. Once the accent was taken away from functional activities, these got worse. This showed that the content of the physical therapy made a difference. Not surprisingly, the physical therapists found that improvement in one area was likely to have a good effect on other areas.

Attenders Did Much Better than Nonattenders

Looking back over the eighteen-month period of the study, the physical therapists were able to see that it was possible to rank the forty participants in order of how much and how little physical therapy they had received.

Group A consisted of the fourteen MS patients who had received the most therapy. Group B consisted of the fourteen patients who had received the least therapy. Both groups were comparable in terms of where they stood on the Kurtzke disability scale at the start of the study.

The results were very encouraging. Although both groups did deteriorate in their range of voluntary movements, patients in group A, who had received the most physical therapy, deteriorated significantly less than those in group B, who had received the least physical therapy.

Physical therapy did not actually prevent deterioration in voluntary range of movements, but it did slow it down. There were also significant differences between the two groups in balance activities and activities of daily living. The group who had the most physical therapy got the most benefit. In activities of daily living, they actually improved their abilities. In functional activities, where there was no marked difference between the two groups, group A still fared better than group B.

Why the Physical Therapy Worked

Postural abnormalities were corrected; abnormal movements were corrected; patients learned or relearned new strategies of movement. The regular exercise maximized the potential of the muscles and meant that the muscles did not stop working, did not stop being used, and so did not atrophy.

Conclusions from the ARMS Physical Therapy Study

- Disability caused by postural deformity or disuse atrophy can be minimized.
- Several movement abnormalities can be prevented or delayed.
- Abilities can be maximized.
- The patients who get the most out of physical therapy are those who
  —are referred early
  —have regular assessments
  —have long-term treatment
  —have regular treatment.
- Without early referral, regular assessments, long-term treat-

ment, or regular treatment, patients' disabilities get worse. These disabilities are secondary handicap caused by misuse and disuse and are not part of the disease process itself.

It's worth repeating—regular exercise can make the difference between the patient retaining his ability to stand or walk or becoming wheelchair-bound.

15

Yoga

Yoga deserves a chapter to itself separate from the exercise chapter because it is more a total philosophy than a simple set of postures or keep-fit exercises. It has as much to do with your whole attitude to life and the way that you breathe as with postures.

Yoga is a unity of the mental and the physical. Done properly, it calms the mind and energizes the body. The body and mind are bound up together and cannot be separated. With a strong sense of purpose, the mind can have a powerful influence on the body.

Hatha yoga is based on the relationship between mind and body. It concentrates on the whole body so, as well as developing physical health, it also promotes mental health.

The word "yoga" comes from the Sanskrit and means "join" or "unite." Hatha yoga is about reaching a balance between the positive and negative within oneself. (Ha—sun (positive); tha—moon (negative).

YOGA AND DIS-EASE

The yogic philosophy is that good health is the natural state for human beings. Good health is when the body and mind are in a state of equilibrium. Illness, or dis-ease, is when the body and mind are out of balance.

There is a natural life force within us all that is trying to do its best to keep us healthy. Yogis say that one does not become ill if one leads a natural life. Even if you have been leading the unhealthy lifestyle of western civilization, the body's healing powers are still there, just waiting to be given a fair chance.

YOGA AND MULTIPLE SCLEROSIS

Since the late 1970s, many people with MS have been doing yoga. The Yoga for Health Foundation in Bedfordshire, England, has done a great deal of work with MS patients, and it has proved of great benefit.

Howard Kent, the director of the Yoga for Health Foundation, has personally helped hundreds of people with MS. Although he has not conducted any sort of scientific trial, Howard Kent is certain that yoga helps MS. He says, "We have evidence that where people are effectively maintaining yoga both mentally and physically, it is rare for us to find deterioration." In an anecdotal way, you will frequently find that someone with MS has become a real devotee of yoga, thanks to the benefits that they have experienced from it.

Yoga has many advantages for someone with MS.

- Yoga may help the body's own self-healing mechanism and may slow down or even halt the disease process.
- Yoga stills the mind.
- Yoga increases energy and counteracts fatigue.
- Yoga lifts the mood and counteracts depression.
- Yoga has a good effect on the functioning of the endocrine glands and the circulatory and respiratory systems and improves well-being.
- Yoga does not require any special equipment and you can practice it daily at home.

Every Breath You Take, Every Move You Make

Correct breathing is one of the most important aspects of yoga. You may think that breathing is something that everyone does naturally. In fact, 99 percent of the population breathe incorrectly, with correspondingly ill effects on their bodies.

Breathing is the most important biological function of the

body. Every other activity of the body is closely connected with breathing. To realize just how important breathing is, remember that you could live for weeks without food, days without water, but only a few minutes without air. Breathing is of primary importance to one's state of health, emotional outlook, and length of life.

Most people in the West take short, rapid, shallow breaths, but it is deep, rhythmic breathing that brings health and energy. Any shock makes people seize up. Notice how you breathe out with a sigh of relief when some ordeal is over. When people are anxious, they tend not to breathe out enough. "I held my breath" is a common phrase for being excited or nervous about something. If you hold your breath often enough or only breathe in a shallow way, your body is not going to get the oxygen it needs for energy.

If the energy is not flowing properly, it will affect both your body and your brain. You will get fatigued easily, and feel run down and depressed. If you are breathing deeply and rhythmically, you will find it hard to be tense at the same time.

Breath is the source of energy. Life is breath.

All forms of mental un-ease or physical dis-ease give themselves away in the way you breathe. Someone with MS may well be breathing incorrectly because of the mental and physical difficulties brought on by the disease. This creates a vicious circle because the breathing difficulties themselves only make those problems worse. The way to stop the vicious circle is to exercise control over your breathing. Fortunately, how you breathe is under your voluntary control.

Yoga is about deep abdominal breathing. In a yoga class, you would be taught to be aware of your diaphragm and to breathe down your abdomen instead of up in your chest. You would learn the essentials of breathing, about the breath of relaxation and the breath of energization. Correct breathing is the foundation on which the other aspects of yoga are based. The best place to learn correct breathing is in a yoga class, under the supervision of a good teacher.

The importance of correct breathing is summed up by Howard Kent:

Effective health, mental and physical, depends upon the ability to breathe naturally in an energizing manner and then, when necessity demands it, to breathe in a relaxed way. Many people can do neither and their lives are then largely led in limbo. As a result, effective opposition to any illness or disability proves impossible and deterioration has to set in. That may sound to be a dogmatic statement, but it is true and identifiable.

Stress and Tension

One of the Catch 22s of MS is that stress and tension probably play some part in bringing on an attack of MS. Once you have MS, however, this in itself creates stress and tension both physically and mentally.

The tension created by having MS can seize up the solar plexus (the network of nerves behind the stomach). This interferes with the movement of the diaphragm, and the body's energy flow is blocked. Yoga relaxes the body, opens up the diaphragm, and frees the energy flow.

Problems with balance and movement will make your body try to compensate by using other muscles. This can create unnatural muscle tensions, which, if they go on for a long time, will lead to spasticity and also affect the functioning of the area around the tense muscles. Once your postural abnormalities have been corrected and you have learned how to relax through correct deep breathing, your body will be able to move more freely.

One of the causes of tension in MS is a profound feeling of self-consciousness about your disabled body. Once you lose this disabling self-consciousness, you will be surprised at how much the condition improves. Spasms, spasticity, and clumsiness are worse when you are anxious and self-conscious. If you don't think about it and can relax, these symptoms are far less pronounced. The practice of yoga can help alleviate both the physical and the mental stresses and tensions.

A Peaceful Mind

Most people's minds are forever buzzing with trivial things. One of the most difficult things to do in yoga is to clear your mind.

The rubbish piles up in your mind and races through your head. Yoga aims to clear the debris from your mind. "Yoga is controlling the activities of the mind," said one of the great Yogis of ancient times.

With a still mind, you can concentrate on what it is you want to achieve. A still mind helps you to be single-minded, and single-mindedness is the best way to achieve your particular goals. With a still mind, you will have inner calm and peace instead of inner turmoil and inner hostilities.

The body's healing process works better when you are in a positive state of mind, and yoga helps you get into a positive state of mind. If your mind is at peace, your body can be used to the best of its ability.

The idea of yoga is to still the mind and be single-minded. It is important to grasp this before doing the exercises, or asanas. "Asana" literally means "holding a position." The asanas are postures in which you can hold your body while at the same time breathing correctly, quieting the mind, and being centered.

Meditation

One way to achieve a calm, still mind is meditation. You clear your mind of daily trivia and concentrate on just one thing. This one thing could be the breath; it could be a "mantra" or chant; it could be a flower. Meditation practiced every day will help you feel calm and refreshed.

Yoga Exercises for MS

People who think of yoga simply as a physical therapy will want to get on to the exercises and to know how these can help them, but the exercises (or asanas) should not be thought of on their own. The correct yoga breathing and the right mental approach are as important as the exercises for your body. Howard Kent calls this the three Bs—brain, breath, and body. He says:

> By the correct use of breathing and mental relaxation I have seen people move legs, with control, which have not moved in years;

I have seen people get up from the floor unaided for the first time in years. Once the inhibitions are removed, the body's real powers can reveal themselves.

Any book on yoga will show you that there is a vast range of yoga exercises or asanas. None of them is harmful to people with MS. To what extent these can be practiced depends on the individual and the degree of disability.

When people with MS first start yoga, they often find it difficult to do a particular movement or hold a position. With practice, however, many people with MS find that they can make dramatic progress, and they discover quite quickly that they can do some exercises they never thought possible.

If you have never done yoga before, it is hard to learn how to do it from a book. It is far better to go to a class. If you go to an ordinary yoga class near where you live, tell the teacher you have MS. You may find that you cannot do some of the balance exercises at first (such as standing on one leg with your hands in a prayer position), but you may well be able to do them with a bit of practice.

For more information, contact:

Yoga Journal
2054 University Avenue
Berkeley, CA 94704
Tel: 415-841-9200

Exercises to Do at Home

Once you have learned some basic exercises in a class, you can do them at home on your own. Ideally, to get the best out of it, you should practice yoga every day for at least fifteen minutes.

Remember that yoga asanas tone up the neuromuscular system of the body and keep it in full working order; they develop and control the respiratory system, increasing oxygen flow and vitality. The internal organs work better, the spine is kept strong and supple, and you enjoy a sense of real well-being.

16

Mental Attitude

Any disability in your body will almost inevitably have some disabling effect on your mind. Your whole identity as a person is bound up with how you feel about yourself. When your body does not do the things it used to do, you are likely to feel worse about yourself.

The trauma of being told that you have MS is made worse by the fact that people think that multiple sclerosis must mean an inevitable downward slide into paralysis and a wheelchair. That scenario is not necessarily true. Everything in this book is based on the real possibility of being able to halt that downward slide of MS if you start a self-help program as soon as possible.

If it is early in your disease and you are not yet noticeably disabled, it is most important that you put in your mind's eye a mental picture of yourself in the future as someone who is healthy, active, and independent. Do not give room in your mind to a future picture of yourself as someone ill, crippled, and with a life that has fallen apart.

The mental pictures you conjure up in your mind are incredibly powerful, without you realizing it. They have a way of being self-fulfilling. Concentrate your mind all the time on being healthy, strong, and active. Will yourself to stay well.

Knowing that there are self-help therapies that work and knowing that there are countless numbers of people with MS who have *improved*, rather than gotten worse, as a result of following particular therapies should make you feel more positive about things. You can hope for the best rather than for the worst.

BODY IMAGE

Unlike people born with a handicap, everyone with MS can easily remember all of the things they could do before they had the disease. Everyone with MS was at one time fit and healthy, able to run around, play sports, sprint to catch a bus, leap up and down stairs, dance, and do all those other things that you take for granted until you find that you can't do them any longer.

When things like that become impossible, your body image changes, sometimes dramatically. People with MS come to see themselves as no longer useful or attractive to others. They must also learn to live with what is still the stigma of MS. A poor self-image can cause them to fear rejection by their partner or prospective partners. Thinking this can cause it to happen.

Despite your symptoms and disabilities, it is important to try to keep hold of a positive body image. MS is no excuse for not taking care of your appearance, even if money is short. Many women I know with MS are beautiful and elegant, even though they may be in a wheelchair or walking with the aid of sticks.

REACTIONS TO MS

The counselor at the ARMS Research Unit, Julia Segal, has compiled a paper called "Reactions to MS" (available from ARMS), gleaned from the experience of ARMS in counseling hundreds of people with MS. Julia Segal concludes:

> There is MS . . . and there is the *reaction to MS*. The reaction to MS can be more destructive than the MS itself. But the reaction to the MS can be affected by support from other people and counselling. People faced with the diagnosis of MS can react in different ways—their strategies for dealing with this disaster can vary.

Denial

One common strategy is denial—if you pretend that you haven't got MS, it will go away. The thought processes of someone who chooses to deny that they have MS will go something like this:

> I don't tell people . . . they couldn't cope with it . . . I couldn't
> cope with their pity . . . I'm afraid if I rest I will never get up
> again . . . people will think I'm lazy . . . I make excuses rather
> than tell people it's MS . . .

A common reason given for the denial approach is that people with MS fear that they will lose their job if their employer finds out that they have MS. This might be a well-founded fear in some cases, although you might be surprised how helpful your employer is.

Another reason that people prefer to sweep their MS under the carpet is because there is still, unfortunately, a fair amount of stigma attached to MS. Once you declare that you have MS, your status as a person in society seems to go down. People do behave toward disabled people differently. Everyone has seen the "Does he take sugar?" kind of behavior, where if you're sitting in a wheelchair people assume that you can't speak for yourself.

Many people with MS lead a sort of double life. They tell some people but not others. They are likely to confide everything to other people with MS and turn to them for support and advice. Yet they may say nothing about their MS to the world at large, their family members, and employers.

With this strategy, there is always the risk of being found out. Also, of course, this only works if your disabilities don't give you away.

Few people like others to feel sorry for them. Once you declare to the world that you have MS, however, people are likely to respond to you with "Oh, poor you!" They are also quite likely to ring up other friends and commiserate about your misfortune: "Isn't it terrible about poor John!" So instead of just being John, or Jane, you are "poor John" in the eyes of others.

Pretending that you haven't got MS is a hard act to keep up because you're always under the strain of hiding something from other people. Even so, there might be some good practical reasons to keep up the pretense until you absolutely must reveal the truth. It's a common strategy for the period after diagnosis,

a sort of holding strategy, until you decide what you're going to do.

Julia Segal, the ARMS counselor, argues that there is a price to pay if you continue to pretend that you haven't got MS. Friends will melt away because it's clear that you didn't trust them; you will find yourself more and more socially isolated, as your attitude may be pushing people away from you. You are denying other people the choice of whether they want to be with you or not. It is very stressful always putting on a pretense. Also, you might be foolishly denying yourself help and support—both practical and emotional—that you really need.

MS as a Whole Identity

The other extreme to denial is letting MS take you over completely so that it dominates your life. There are some people for whom multiple sclerosis becomes their whole identity. They have MS, but MS also has them.

After diagnosis, such people succumb to MS completely. They may give up work; they may go on disability pension; they may apply for a disabled sticker; they join some MS club; they meet other people less and less. They shift their whole life to a subculture of disabled people. MS becomes their hobby. They have no others.

Needing to meet and talk to other people with MS may be a very important stage that newly diagnosed people have to go through. Making MS your whole life, however, can create problems with families and friends.

I vividly remember the story of a man with MS who lived, breathed, and slept MS. It was all he ever thought about or talked about. One day his wife screamed at him, "If I ever hear the words MS again in this house I shall go stark staring mad!" This was a sufficient jolt for him to put MS into the context of his whole life and lead a more balanced existence.

MS has become part of your life, but it is not your whole life. Dominate it before it dominates you.

MS as an Excuse

Another strategy that I have noticed in quite a few people with MS is using MS as an excuse for opting out of life as it should be lived. For example, a friend asks you to go out for a day in the country. You say, "Sorry, I can't, I've got MS." You really want to go, but you fear that your MS symptoms will make the day problematic. MS *does* get in the way. The symptoms are real, but some of the fears about the symptoms make them severe only in your head. By using MS as an excuse, you are denying yourself many opportunities to have a nice, or interesting, or pleasurable time.

Depression

Depression is a much more common reaction to a diagnosis of MS than euphoria, which has been said to go with having MS. Depression is most likely to happen soon after diagnosis, when the full implications of the disease hit you. If you have seen people in advanced stages of the disease or you have read medical textbooks about MS, you may fear that the worst is going to happen to you and so become awash with gloom and despair.

Depression is particularly bad for someone with MS because it weakens an already weakened immune system. Your state of mind has a direct effect on your state of health.

It is not easy to counteract depression, but one Australian woman I know succeeds in keeping depression at bay with a simple five-point plan.

1. Get plenty of sleep. Never get over-tired. (Notice how much more depressed and irritable you feel when you are tired.)
2. Eat often and plenty. Never allow yourself to get weak with hunger.
3. Exercise at least once a day. Exercise boosts your circulation, gets oxygen into your brain, and stokes up the body chemistry so that endorphins—the well-being hormones—are released.
4. Always have something to look forward to. Having MS can

be like living in a dark tunnel. Always have treats in store to bring some sunshine into your life.

5. Be sociable. Take an interest in other people. This takes your mind off you and your troubles. Having MS is not a sentence to social isolation.

Add to that list:

6. Think positively.
7. Take care to look good. You can only feel good about yourself if you feel you look good.
8. Stick to as ordered a routine as you can and keep on top of things. That way you know where you are.
9. Keep your mind active and interested.
10. Do something that gives you a sense of achievement, for example, a creative hobby or helping other people in the community. Being proud of what you do is a great booster to the spirits.
11. Live in the present and get the most out of each experience as it is actually happening. Do not dwell on the past or be fearful about the future.

Some people have actually felt that getting MS is a blessing in disguise. Sometimes such people are religious. For them, having MS has made them truly appreciate some things in life that they used to take for granted. These are the people who derive new-found joy from the scent of a flower or the beauty of a tree. They strip from their lives all the nonsense that clutters up most people's daily existence, and instead just concentrate on the truly important things.

Life is lived slowly but richly. People who are able to rush because they can move fast miss the beauty of the rose petals. However, most people with MS would prefer to be able to move fast, given the choice.

Self-esteem

Self-esteem is your most vital asset. MS can dent it more visibly than a limp in your walk. The most off-putting thing to other people is not that you walk with a limp or drag your left foot, but that you look downcast, grim-faced, embittered, or ready to bite anyone's head off if they speak to you.

Of course, when you have MS, it is easy to feel damaged, a psychological as well as a physical cripple, a second-rate person. This negative attitude is probably that most disabling thing of all. It is vital to fight it off.

Self-esteem is so important because people always think of you the same way you think of yourself. If you lack self-respect, you will not win respect from other people. If you are filled with self-loathing, you can be sure of a few enemies. If you have no love for yourself, no one else will be able to love you either. This is one of the hardest facts of life—but true.

Negative Thoughts and Feelings

Negative thoughts and feelings are known to undermine the health, lower the body's resistance to infection, and delay the healing process. A negative personality is one who is lacking in self-confidence and full of self-doubt. Negative people say "no" rather than "yes." They say "I can't" rather than "I can." They always imagine the most pessimistic outcome of any event. They are afraid of everything. They have no faith in their own powers, so they always go to other people for help. They tend to fail because they have an attitude that says "it can't work." They tend to see the worst in everything and everybody. They are very good at complaining and at forecasting doom and gloom.

Many people will hate to admit that they recognize themselves or some of themselves some of the time in this portrait. A negative personality, who only has negative thoughts and feelings, cannot be happy. Not only will such a person be unhappy, he or she will also be unwell, as this kind of negative programming is incompatible with good health.

You know from your own experience how emotions can affect your body. Winning something makes you feel on top of the world, whereas bad news makes you feel ill, with perhaps symptoms of sickness, palpitations, a dry mouth, weakness, and so on.

The negative emotions all have a bad effect on your health. Rage, fear, grief, sorrow, fright, jealousy, despondency, or pessimism make you feel bad physically. Of these, fear is supposed to be the most noxious. On the other hand, the positive emotions of love, joy, and compassion make you feel good physically.

When you're told you have MS it is almost impossible to avoid feeling a wide range of negative emotions. Fear, grief, anger, rage, terror, shock, and bewilderment are all common feelings, particularly at the beginning.

A sense of loss is very common after you have been told that you have MS. It is as if part of you has died, and you naturally mourn and grieve for it. The period of bereavement for your old self will take time, but the fear may linger.

If negative feelings and emotions are getting the better of you, seek help. Bottling things up will only make things worse. There are various ways to help shift your emphasis away from the negative and toward the positive. These include yoga, meditation, visualization, psychotherapy, and counseling.

Visualization

Visualization techniques have become well known through the work of the Simontons in the USA, who have been using them to good effect in cancer treatment. Cancer patients are told to imagine things like white knights (white blood cells) killing the evil cancer cells.

It would be possible to use similar techniques in multiple sclerosis. The mind is very powerful, and the mental images that you conjure up in your head can be translated into real life.

The best position for visualization is sitting erect (if possible) and breathing deeply. How you imagine your MS being overcome is up to you. Perhaps instead of conjuring up the image of the body's troops driving out the enemy, you may prefer to imagine pictures of yourself. In your mind's eye, always picture yourself happy, healthy, and active. You could imagine yourself swimming, or running along a beautiful beach, or disco dancing, or climbing mountains, or whatever.

This technique of intensely imagining yourself doing something active has worked in some cancer cases. It is also a technique used more and more to achieve success in competitive sport—players go through the mental process of, say, scoring a goal. Once you've rehearsed something carefully in your mind, it's much more likely to happen in real life. Don't allow room in your head for pictures of yourself in worse condition than you are now.

Fears

ARMS counselor Julia Segal has found that everyone with MS has a different worst fear about MS and that talking your fears over with a trained counselor is the best way of dealing with them. In her paper "Reactions to MS," she listed some of the things that people fear most.

- being in a wheelchair
- nobody finding you attractive any more
- being totally paralyzed
- being cut off from everyone
- going blind and being alone in the dark
- waking up one morning unable to move

With counseling, it is possible to talk these fears through and realize that there is a less stark side to each of these scenarios. First, it hasn't happened yet and might never happen. Second, the fears themselves are probably unrealistic. For example, men do still flirt with women in wheelchairs if they have attractive personalities and take pride in their appearance.

COUNSELING

Counseling really can help. People can be helped to feel and behave better. Anxieties are brought out into the open and can be controlled with the help of a trained counselor. It is very important that people with MS feel that they have someone to turn to.

Counseling for someone with MS can help in the following ways:

* Work with a counselor can reestablish the ability to enjoy life. The counselor can help deal with the anger that is preventing recognition of real pleasures and remaining abilities.
* Counseling can uncover hidden love. Resentment and anger arising out of the MS can cover up and bury real love and affection. Counseling can help people to find, recognize, and express their love again.
* Counseling can sometimes help lift depression and stop the person with MS from seeming to punish the family, and so making them feel guilty.

Counselors in the United States

Some chapters of the national MS Society have peer counselors. For more information call the MS Society's Information Resource Center at 1-800-227-3166, 11 a.m. to 6 p.m., Mondays through Fridays.

Talking things over with the telephone counselors can help people sort things out, which makes them feel better. Sometimes talking to a completely anonymous person, just a voice on the telephone, is easier than talking to someone in the family, because they may be involved in the problem themselves.

The Metaphysics of Illness

Some psychologists think that each physical illness has a mental cause; each physical illness has a particular attitude or set of attitudes that go to make up the personality of the person who has that illness. Nowadays, "the cancer personality" is a phrase that people understand.

In the United States, the metaphysics of illness has quite a following. One of the handbooks of this approach is *Heal Your Body* by Louise L. Hay.* For each physical condition, she lists a probable metaphysical cause, and the new thought pattern that will overcome the problem.

PROBLEM	PROBABLE CAUSE	NEW THOUGHT PATTERN
Multiple sclerosis	Mental hardness, hard-heartedness, iron will, inflexibility	I no longer try to control; I flow along with the joy of life.

Louise Hay has since written *You Can Heal Your Life* (published by Hay House, USA) in which she describes how changing your thought patterns can, literally, heal you.

A similar metaphysical approach is taken by the American authors of *Health for the Whole Person* published by Westview Press (editors Hastings, Fadiman, and Gordon). A person with MS is described as having the following attitude:

> This person feels forced to undertake some kind of physical activity and does not want to. He has to work without help, has to support himself and usually others. He does not want to, and wishes help or support.

You might feel that neither of these descriptions of an "MS attitude" accurately describes yourself. Even so, you might feel that examining your thought processes and attitudes to see whether they need changing is a worthwhile thing to do.

---

*Published by Louise L. Hay, 11906 Goshen Avenue, Los Angeles, CA 90049.

17

Hints on Daily Living

MS symptoms can come and go, even within one day. Sometimes it seems that there is neither rhyme nor reason why you should feel worse today than you did yesterday. However, there are some things that can bring on MS symptoms and so should be avoided as much as possible. These include humid heat, hot baths, over-exertion, stressful events, over-tiredness, and hunger. In this chapter, I discuss these triggers.

This chapter also gives hints on how to deal with some of the unwanted symptoms of MS that affect daily life, such as fatigue, constipation, and incontinence. I also explain why habits such as drinking and smoking are so bad for you when you have MS.

When you have MS, you should try to do everything to maintain the best health possible. The diet and exercise advice already given would help that, but nutrition and exercise alone are not enough.

HOMEOSTASIS

One of the oldest concepts of good health, going back to the time of Hippocrates, is homeostasis. Nowadays we might call this balance or harmony. What quite quickly becomes apparent once you have MS is that your area of homeostasis shrinks.

Before you had MS, you could probably tolerate extremes of temperature without too much complaint; you could probably tolerate a humid summer; you could probably go Christmas shopping without flaking out; you could probably work long hours when you needed to without feeling like a radio with run-down batteries. Once you have MS, however, you look at other people and marvel at what they can do. They have the health and energy to do things that seem impossible to you now.

The area within which healthy people still feel healthy and energetic is considerably greater than that for most people with MS. In other words, what will maintain homeostasis in a healthy person is not what will maintain homeostasis in someone with MS. (See Figure 15.)

The possibilities do become limited. The kind of work that you do, your family commitments, how you get around, where you live, where you go on holiday, and what type of holiday you have are all quite seriously affected by having MS.

FIGURE 15
Homeostasis

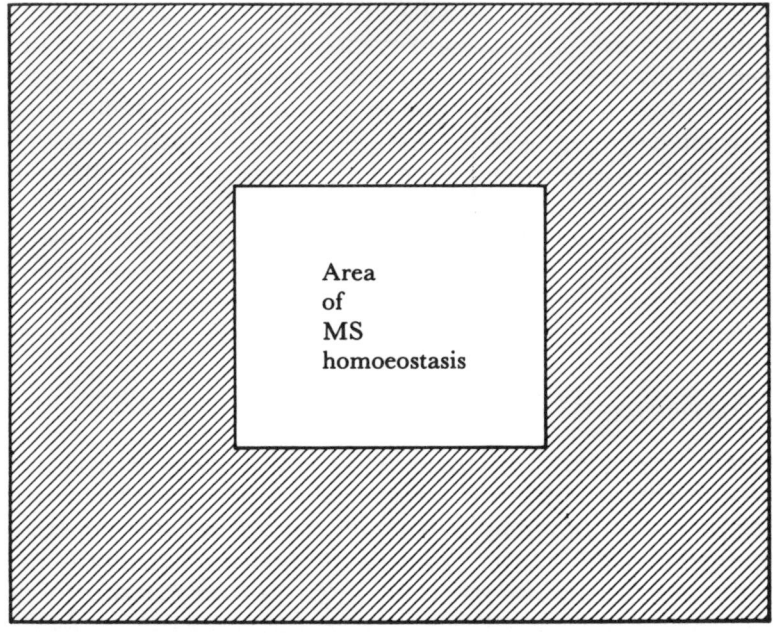

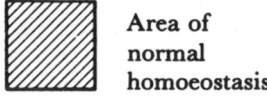 Area of normal homoeostasis

You have to find out for yourself what conditions will maintain your homeostasis and what circumstances are dangerously outside it. These will differ from person to person.

For example, I know that for me the ideal temperature to maintain my own homeostasis is around 658F, with no humidity. Once it goes above 758F, with any humidity, I feel like the proverbial wet dishcloth and cannot function properly.

I have had to impose similar limits regarding how far I can drive in one trip, how many hours I can work, how late I can stay up, etc. My own limited sphere of homeostasis corresponds roughly with the small box in Figure 15. The old me, pre-MS, could operate very well within the bigger box.

I do find that I can remain stable as long as I stay within this small box. The trouble starts when I try to go beyond it.

FATIGUE

Fatigue is one of the most insidious symptoms of MS and one that has devastating effects in almost every area of life. Fatigue may make it impossible for you to carry on working full time; it makes it more difficult to bring up a family.

Fatigue in MS is not like normal fatigue, from which you can recuperate quite easily with a good rest. It is chronic fatigue, where everything seems to be an effort. Even simple things, like hanging out the washing, become daunting tasks.

Fatigue in MS is not just tired muscles. It is the effect of the disease on the nerves that go to the muscles and also the effect of the disease on the sensory nerves. The sensory nerves transmit touch, sight, taste, smell, and hearing. So, when you get fatigued, you can sometimes experience blurring of vision or slurring of speech.

What happens when you get fatigued can differ from person to person. Fatigue often worsens existing symptoms or brings on symptoms that only happen when you are fatigued. Also, old symptoms can come back, with the nasty habit of reminding you of your last attack. Severe fatigue can also bring on episodes of vertigo, where the ceiling spins. You can also feel ill, as if you have the flu.

There are certain things that can bring on fatigue, as well as other MS symptoms. When you know what these things are, fatigue is easier to avoid.

What brings on fatigue can differ from person to person. However, some of the most common things are a hot day, humid weather, a hot bath, over-exertion, over-tiredness, a heavy meal, smoking, and stress. Fatigue can also be one of the major symptoms of a food allergy.

Why Do You Get Fatigued?

Any movement of any muscle requires energy. Energy comes from glucose, and to convert glucose into energy the muscle needs oxygen.

Oxygen is brought to the muscle by the blood circulating through it. If there is not enough oxygen because of poor circulation, substances like lactic acid accumulate and prevent the muscles from working. The oxygen supply to the muscles is increased when the blood flow is improved by exercise.

Of course, the whole process of energy production and muscle contraction is highly complex. However, it is important to understand the essential link between blood flow, oxygen, and the working of the muscles. Fatigue happens when the blood flow (hence, the oxygen flow to the muscles) is inadequate.

Exercise to Combat Fatigue

If you are physically fit, you have a better chance of withstanding fatigue. To keep fit, you must keep the muscles exercised. You should never exercise to the point of exhaustion and should stop before feeling tired or hot. However, if you do not do any exercise at all, you will get fatigued much more easily than if you do.

Exercise tones up the whole system (see Chapter 14). After a session of gym, yoga, or swimming, for example, you should have more energy, not less. Your body will give you early warning signals as to when it is time to stop and rest.

HEAT AND HUMIDITY

A common experience with MS is to become very sensitive to heat, particularly humid heat. Hot, humid summers can be hell for someone with MS, who feels weak and drained all the time with no energy for anything.

It is important to keep cool. Air conditioning would be very nice if you could afford it. A fan in every room is a second best.

Dry heat seems to be tolerated by people with MS, and many enjoy being in not too hot sunshine, as long as there is no humidity. Where you choose to go for your holiday becomes an issue. It may be better to go on holiday off-season, when it is not too hot.

Be very careful with hot baths. They can bring on MS symptoms very rapidly, as well as leaving you very weak. These symptoms tend to go away once the effects of the hot bath have worn off but are unpleasant nevertheless. They can be avoided by making sure that the bath water is comfortably warm but not hot.

OVER-EXERTION

One of the problems about having MS is that many people—particularly those who are young and energetic—want to prove that they can still do all the things they used to do. So they overcompensate, and make themselves ill by over-exertion.

Young people with MS who have not told their employer, their workmates, or even their family are more at risk of over-exertion. Driving a lorry from London to Scotland in one haul may be fine if you are a fit and healthy man, but it's simply asking for trouble if you have MS and are hiding it from everyone.

The ones who seem to suffer most from over-exertion are wives. Women stricken with MS have, in my view, the toughest time. In our so-called emancipated society, they are expected to do three full-time jobs: go out to work, run the household, and be a mother. The energy available when you have MS is not enough to fulfill even one of these roles properly, let alone three.

I have received letters from wives that have made my blood boil. Even though the wife has MS, the husband still expects her to cook, clean, look after the children, *and* go out to work to help earn a living.

Time and time again, women in that situation are called "lazy" if they do not visibly do all the chores. A woman with MS may feel so weak after a day at work that she is only fit to slump in the armchair. Not wanting to be labeled "lazy" or "selfish," many of these women force themselves to cook a meal, clean the house, do the laundry and the ironing, or whatever. The kind of chores that women are expected to do are particularly energy-consuming. The easiest place to suffer from over-exertion is in the home. Fatigue is the likely result.

Many women suffer this kind of unfair treatment from their families because they may *look* perfectly OK. The "invisible" symptoms of MS, such as fatigue, are not obvious to other people in the same way that a limp or a hacking cough would be.

Continual over-exertion such as this can only lead to trouble; worsening symptoms are almost inevitable as there is no rest from the constant strain.

The workload simply must be shared with other people or lessened, or both. This kind of situation may require relationship counseling or help from the social services, if you can get it.

MS will almost certainly mean altering the traditional roles in your household, and this will take time to adjust.

WORK

Over-exertion is often tied up with the work you do. Many people find that their job is simply not compatible with having MS. For example, a surveyor could not continue to climb up on roofs or balance along parapet walls. Two journalists I know could not keep on rushing about everywhere and meeting tight deadlines; a pilot I knew had to forget about flying planes. The list is endless.

Once you have MS, your "energy cake" is much smaller, and

you have to choose how you are going to share it out. It probably means setting your sights lower. It will probably mean watching your contemporaries being promoted over your head, when you can see that—if things had turned out differently—it could have been you being promoted.

One of the most painful things about MS is that it does strike young people in their prime. This is just the age when people are aiming to make it in their chosen career or walk of life. It hurts to see success, and probably fortune too, being snatched from your grasp. This is particularly so at a period when someone's whole identity—male or female—is so bound up with the work they do.

Even if you succeed in not getting worse, even if you successfully stabilize the disease, you will probably still have to sacrifice some work. If your present job is strenuous and stressful, you will have to decide whether the price you will have to pay in fatigue is worth it. If you continue to work full-time in a demanding job, you may be too tired to do anything else when you come home. The idea is probably to find some suitable part-time work, if possible, or change to a less demanding job that is full-time, even if it means stepping down a few rungs in the career ladder.

You do not have to give up work altogether because you have MS. It would probably be pretty damaging to your self-esteem and self-confidence—as well as to your pocket—if you did. Try to find the right balance between work and the rest of your life.

OVER-TIREDNESS

If you feel tired (not the same as fatigue), then rest. If you don't rest, your tiredness may turn into fatigue all too easily.

A rest at some time during the day is highly desirable. If you can manage twice a day, so much the better. Resting will feel like recharging your batteries. You don't have to go to sleep. Just lie down and relax completely. You could read a book or meditate. You will feel more relaxed if you put your feet up.

SLEEP

If you are going short of sleep, you are bound to feel fatigued. Try to go to bed early.

Tell yourself that you will be in bed by a particular time every night, with perhaps one late night. This means being firm with other people. If you are invited out anywhere, politely insist on leaving when you feel that it is time for you to go. Doubtless, your host or hostess will make you feel guilty about leaving so "early," but guilt is better than fatigue.

If you can manage it, get some sleep during the day. An hour or so after lunch is usually the best time. Some symptoms of MS go away almost miraculously after a good sleep.

EATING

A woman with MS gave me some invaluable advice that works like magic in some instances of fatigue—eat and drink plenty and often. Being "weak with hunger" has a particular relevance to people with MS. The symptoms of that unnatural fatigue (what some people call "feeling MSy") creep over you when you begin to feel hungry, and get worse as you get hungrier. If you go without breakfast, you could be feeling deathly by mid-morning.

Of all the things that bring on fatigue, this is the easiest to overcome. At home, you have instant access to the fridge or pantry (stick to nutritious snacks, not junk food). Problems arise when you go out. Some people serve dinner late, and your legs could be like jelly by the time the soup is served. Far better to eat a little something before you leave the house. If you're going on a journey, take emergency rations with you.

There's no need to stuff yourself, or get fat; simply plug the hole in your stomach before you get really hungry and weak.

How to Eat Properly

Eating properly may sound trivial, but it is in fact vitally important to good health. Here are some general guidelines:

1. Chew All of Your Food Slowly and Thoroughly.
In chewing, your teeth tear your food apart, and the food mixes with saliva in your mouth, which is the first stage in the digestive process. It is not good to swallow lots of unchewed food, as it gives the digestive substances a hard time. The more thoroughly you chew, the greater the amount of nutrients your body will absorb. Semi-digested food particles passing through the intestinal wall may be involved in allergic reactions and other symptoms of ill health.

2. Ideally, Do Not Drink with Meals.
Too much fluid with food interferes with the digestive substances. Ideally, do not drink any fluids from at least half an hour before any meal until half an hour after that meal.

3. Drink at Least Five Glasses of Water a Day.
When you are thirsty, drink water in preference to anything else. Go for pure bottled still spring water or filtered tap water. Still water is better than the artificially carbonated waters. Do not drink ice cold water.

4. Rotate Your Foods.
Food rotation means eating a particular food only once in every four days. This applies particularly to the grains containing gluten, which are wheat, barley, oats, and rye.

A seasonal diet, of foods eaten only in season, would be ideal to keep our bodies attuned and allow recovery time for the digestive enzymes. Of course, this is virtually impossible today.

A break of four days between foods gives the liver time to process any toxin from a food group and the enzymes time to recuperate fully. By rotating foods, you are assured of fully digesting the food you take in, leading to less toxic waste.

5. Attempt to Eat in a Biochemical Balance.
Aim for a biochemical balance between acid and alkaline foods and between cooked and raw foods. You might need a macrobiotic cookbook to help you discover which foods are acid and

which are alkaline. If you choose foods from opposite polarities, it helps the body stay balanced.

6. Food Combining for Health.
Ideally, do not eat protein with starches, and do not eat fruit with protein meals. There are several books about food combining that explain its health benefits.

Weight

Despite the advice about eating when hungry, it is sensible to lose weight if you are overweight. If you are carrying around surplus weight, you will get fatigued more quickly.

Food Allergies

Fatigue is one of the classic symptoms of food allergies. Ironically, the time when you are most likely to get symptoms from an allergic food is *not* just after eating the offending food but when you have not eaten the offending food for a while. This would tie in with fatigue symptoms coming on when you are hungry. This is called a "masked allergy." Some people find that their fatigue disappears once they have identified and excluded the foods to which they are allergic. (See Chapter 9.)

SMOKING

Smoking has very bad effects on MS. It can cause worsening of MS symptoms. One of the frequent effects of smoking is to lower skin temperature. This can aggravate MS, in which people tend to suffer from a feeling of cold in the hands and feet anyway. Also, eye problems in MS can sometimes be associated with smoking.

Everyone knows that smoking can cause lung cancer, bronchitis and emphysema, and cardiovascular disorders. The toxic substances from a single cigarette, such as cadmium, lower the blood level of vitamin C and destroy about 25 mg of the vitamin.

Smoking can only do you harm. It is one of the greatest health hazards and the most preventable cause of premature death. Smoking also interferes with the beneficial effects of a diet high in essential fatty acids.

So, *don't smoke.*

DRINKING ALCOHOL

Alcohol can worsen MS symptoms, which can make you look like a drunk anyway. Alcohol can make coordination worse and may affect standing, walking, finger movements, eye movements, and speech. Far from being a stimulant, alcohol acts as a depressant. It could well make you feel low rather than high.

In some diets for MS (for example, the Swank Diet), alcohol is allowed in *small quantities.* If you find that a glass of good wine or sherry does not make you feel ill, there's no harm in drinking them occasionally.

However, a lot of alcohol can do you harm. It inhibits the conversion process of the essential fatty acids, and nothing should get in the way of this vital process.

Alcohol causes the amount of saturated fat in the blood to increase. It increases the need for vitamin B_1, pantothenic acid, and choline.

Be careful in case you have an allergy to some of the ingredients in alcoholic drinks. Sugar is added to many alcoholic drinks. Yeast is added to some.

Alcohol is probably the most difficult thing to refuse socially. Everyone expects everyone else to drink, and a glass of something is always being shoved in your hand at parties. However, if drink does make you feel ill, you must resist this kind of pressure. Insist on mineral water or pure unsweetened fruit juices.

CONSTIPATION

Constipation is a common complaint in MS. It is important to find a remedy because continued constipation has many bad effects. There is a build-up of toxins in the system; the full bowel presses on the bladder and makes you more likely to be incontinent; you feel uncomfortable.

Fiber

The ARMS EFA diet (Chapter 6) is high in fiber, or roughage. High fiber foods include onions, parsnips, celery, peas, beans, stringy vegetables—all raw or lightly cooked; whole grains, whole wheat bread; bran; oatmeal; nuts; and fresh and dried fruits. The ARMS diet also recommends additional bran to be sprinkled on breakfast cereals, fruit purées, low fat yogurts, etc. Refined foods are low in fiber and can only make constipation worse, not better.

Psyllium Seed Husks

Another excellent fiber is psyllium seed husks. These are a valuable source of nondigestible plant fiber. As much as one tablespoon can be taken with each meal until bowel regulation occurs. The amount can then be reduced to one or two teaspoons, three times a day, every fourth day (to rotate this fiber with other fiber foods on a four-day rotation basis). Psyllium seed husks are available from drugstores.

Water

When you are eating a high fiber diet, it is most important to drink a lot of water. The fiber needs the water to pass easily along the bowel.

If fact, water is probably the most important anti-constipation agent. The first thing to do if you are not regular is to drink as much water as possible. Make a habit of drinking one glassful when you get up.

Evening Primrose Oil

Many people have found that their constipation has been relieved after taking evening primrose oil capsules. The frequent use of oils like sunflower seed oil in salad dressing and cooking will help, too.

Dried Fruit

Another tip is to chew whole fruit and dried fruit such as figs and take linseeds and/or stewed prunes before each meal.

Acidophilus

New research into intestinal flora ("probiotics") has found that bowel regularity has more to do with your intenstinal flora than with the amount of fiber you eat. Many people swear by taking capsules of acidophilus, a friendly bacteria found in the gut. This bacteria would be decimated if you were taking antibiotics.

Vitamin C

A good intake of vitamin C helps keep the stools soft—as much as 2 to 4 grams, three times a day. The use of vitamin C as a bowel softener has considerable value beyond the retention of fluid in the colon. It also serves as a detoxifying substance for toxins formed by bacteria in the colon.

Exercise

If you are sagging in your posture and sluggish generally, you are more likely to be constipated. Toning up the whole system by exercise will get you going in more ways than one.

Do not take laxatives. This makes the bowel lazy. It also means that your body loses much-needed vitamins and minerals. Continued use of laxatives can make you feel very unwell.

Finally, allow enough unhurried time on the toilet.

To sum up, combat constipation with

- a high fiber diet including added bran
- lots of water—start the day with a glass of water

- oils such as evening primrose oil or sunflower seed oil
- lots of whole fruit and dried fruits like figs
- linseeds and/or stewed prunes before each meal
- acidophilus capsules once a day
- unhurried time on the toilet

BLADDER PROBLEMS

Of all symptoms of MS, incontinence is probably the one people feel most miserable about. When there is damage to the nerve pathways in the lower part of the spine, control of the bladder can be weakened. You may feel an urgent need to go to the toilet frequently, even though there is not much urine in the bladder.

Alternatively, some people suffer from bladder retention, when they cannot pass water, no matter how hard they try or how much they feel that they want to go. In more advanced cases of MS, double incontinence (fecal incontinence) can sometimes happen too.

These are particularly distressing symptoms because they are surrounded in our society by feelings of embarrassment and shame. Some people with MS find the possibility of wetting themselves in public, not being able to find a toilet in time, or emitting an unpleasant odor to be a worse handicap than, say, walking with a limp.

The present-day statistics are that 50 to 80 percent of all MS patients experience bladder problems at some point. However, there are many anecdotal cases of bladder symptoms clearing up when people have detected their food allergies and cut out the offending foods. Hyperbaric oxygen also helps bladder symptoms in some people.

You may find that, if you stick to the self-help management program in this book, you may not suffer from bladder problems at all. I have never suffered from any bladder problems myself (knock on wood!)

Bladder symptoms often become worse than they need to be because of simple neglect. A consultant/urologist speaking at a recent symposium on MS said, "I am sad to say that some of the greatest cases of neglect have been those with neuropathic disorders." He was talking about MS specifically.

Patients may feel embarrassed to seek help about something still considered vaguely shameful. And doctors may not be referring patients to the right kind of help early enough.

Here again, we have a situation similar to that of secondary handicap. Contractures and deformities can happen to someone with MS, not as part of the disease process, but because they did not receive physical therapy early enough. Likewise, many people with MS put up with agonizing symptoms, such as bladder urinary retention, when the right help could have saved them pain and misery. Bladder infections can be a secondary complication of bladder problems. With the right help early enough, these can be avoided.

Secondary complications should never be allowed to happen. It is most important to deal with bladder problems like retention and infection before they can lead to anything worse. There is now something called CISC—clean intermittent self-catheterization—for patients who are not able to empty their bladders properly.

For the whole range of bladder symptoms, there is a range of drugs available on prescription from your doctor. So you should see your doctor and ideally ask to be referred to a consultant urologist at the nearest hospital where they have one. Some urology departments have incontinence counselors. With the help of drugs, possibly a catheter, possibly HBO, possibly special pants and pads, it is possible to manage the problem of incontinence in such a way as to lead a nearly normal life.

Drinking

You might think that, if you cut down on your fluid intake, your need to rush to the toilet will be reduced. Not so. The trouble with drinking very little is that the urine becomes concentrated and smelly, which can create its own problems.

Ideally you should drink at least five glasses of fluid a day, more (eight to ten) if possible. Drink more earlier in the day. Do not drink anything for a couple of hours before going to bed if you normally have to get up in the night to go to the toilet. That way, you are less likely to be up several times in the night. If you wear a catheter, it is very important to drink a lot of fluid; otherwise, the catheter may collect debris. A high fluid intake will prevent this.

Drinking a good amount is also an essential to avoid constipation. In fact, constipation itself can be a cause of stress incontinence because the full bowel is pressing on the bladder (see section on constipation).

Both coffee and red wine can irritate the bladder lining and make you feel more of an urge to pass water than you would feel otherwise. Other alcoholic drinks could have the same effect too.

Going to the Toilet

It is common sense to organize your life so that you are not far away from a toilet. Before setting out on a journey or going somewhere you have never been before, it is a wise precaution to find out where the toilets are. You might prefer to avoid, for example, motorways that have no service stations on them.

Once in the toilet, make sure that you empty your bladder completely. Stay there long enough to make sure there is nothing left. Women should lean forward to help empty the bladder thoroughly.

STRESS

Some doctors believe that trauma triggers MS in susceptible people. If you ask people with MS where they experienced their first symptom, many will describe a part of the body that suffered a trauma previous to the onset of MS.

Other people will say that there were very stressful events just before MS was diagnosed. Attacks, or relapses, of MS can often be caused by stress.

One definition of stress is not having the resources to meet the demands made on you. The more feeble your resources, the more stressful are demands on you. The more abundant your resources, the less stressful are demands on you.

Resources mean both practical resources, such as money and equipment, and inner resources, such as strength of will and health. Obviously, if you are ill your inner resources will be depleted, and demands that would not feel like stress to a well person suddenly become stressful. The more you can retain or regain your health and well-being, the better you will be able to deal with stress.

Attitude is also very important. Remember that one person's stress is another person's challenge. Your personality, or how you respond to a particular situation, is perhaps more relevant than the stressor itself. For example, some people get a thrill from taking off in an airplane, while others find it stressful. Some people people love working to deadlines, while others seize up at the thought of it.

If you can gain some insight into yourself and see that stress is making your symptoms worse, you could do two things. You could set about reducing these stresses from your life, or you could change your attitude to them (or both).

Many people with MS identify themselves as having very short fuses. Their ability to withstand even minor stress is diminished. If you can see that your reaction to stress is very pronounced, you might benefit from counseling or psychotherapy.

When you feel under stress, the hormones in your body become unbalanced. Cortisol, the hormone of hopelessness and helplessness, interferes with the metabolism of essential fatty acids. So you should try to relax or reduce the circumstances that make you feel stressed.

18

Relationships and Sex

Once you have MS, your relationships with everyone change—including your relationship with yourself. You are the one you have to go on living with, and you have to like your own company first before relationships will work with other people.

Having MS will affect your relationship with yourself, your relationship with your partner if you have one, and your ability to find a partner if you do not have one already.

Having MS will affect your relationships inside the family—with your children if you are a parent and with your parents if you are the "child" with MS. Brothers, sisters, and wider family will also be affected. So will friends, neighbors, colleagues at work, and employers if you have them. The ripples from having MS spread far and wide.

The ideal is that your MS is controlled and never gets bad. The trouble with MS, however, is that people with the disease live with the fear that deterioration is lurking around the next corner. Even if you are only mildly disabled, the fact that you have MS is bound to affect all relationships—if you let it.

Perhaps the most damaging thing that MS can do is to make you feel bad about yourself. This is pernicious because the way you feel about yourself is crucial to having both rewarding relationships and a fulfilling sex life.

RELATIONSHIPS WITH A PARTNER

If you already have an intimate and loving relationship with your partner, there is no reason why MS should threaten the relationship; indeed, it could well bring you closer together. On the other hand, a chronic and potentially disabling illness like MS can throw a severe strain on a relationship that lacks deep intimacy and communication. If the person with MS finds it difficult to talk freely and difficult to accept help or is very demanding or if the partner is unable to offer help, a marriage could be in dire straits.

When either a husband or a wife gets MS, it is difficult to carry on with family life as if nothing has happened. On the other hand, the person with MS does not want to be labeled as an invalid and give up the role of wife, mother, husband, father, or breadwinner.

Even though your body image may have changed, you are still you. You are still able to give and receive love, to laugh, cry, share emotions, and be needed by your family, friends, and colleagues. You will feel more of a sense of worth if you keep reminding yourself that you are needed, loved, and lovable.

If you go round being a misery and a grump, you will find it difficult to like yourself, and you can hardly expect others to like you either. A frown puts people off, but a smile attracts.

You can control your moods if you decide to. It is better to try to take a light-hearted approach to MS problems than a heavy-handed, gloomy one. Certainly, they are no joke, but the people I know with MS who can manage to make a joke out of their difficulties tend to get on much better in life than those who do not. They are the kind who might chuckle, "Oh! There I go, knocking things over again," rather than being embarrassed about it.

Relationship Problems

It is easy to turn MS into the scapegoat for all marital and sexual problems, when it is the basic relationship itself that is at fault. Even so, MS will dramatically affect any relationship. Feelings that neither of you may have had to confront before are likely to hit you with a terrible impact: feelings of fear, frustration, rage, and perhaps hostility and guilt.

Each couple must work out for themselves the issues of dependence and independence—to what extent the one with MS can make demands on the other and to what extent the one without MS should give help to the other. Some sufferers will fall into the "sick" role and use it to manipulate their partners or other relatives, but this will only make them feel guilt and hostility.

These issues are very hard to deal with, but they must be confronted and talked through. It may be necessary to get help from a professional therapist or counselor.

CHILDREN

Children can be very bewildered and shocked by a parent who gets MS. They may have had a mommy who used to run round the park with them or a dad who played football but cannot any longer.

What and when you tell them depends on their age, but the key is to be honest. Try not to tell a four-year-old more than he can understand. Instinctively, children are aware that something is wrong and that you are worried. You need to be aware of this and understand that their behavior can sometimes be disturbed. They need comfort and reassurance. Your children may have to alter their views about what mothers and fathers are supposed to be like, and this adjustment will take time.

Older children may appear outwardly calm or even indifferent when they are told that you have MS, yet inwardly they could be acutely anxious about it. The way to deal with this is to talk to them, giving a little information at a time rather than one long talk. Treat them as adults, and let them play a responsible part in family life.

Children's Fears

Children can feel afraid if one of their parents has MS, but this fear may not be at the conscious level, says ARMS counselor Julia Segal. The deep-down terror is that their mom or dad is going to die because of MS and that they themselves will get MS.

Children can also feel guilty that somehow they were responsible for their parents' MS, particularly if the first attack happened soon after their own birth. Children do feel responsible for their parents; they may well feel that they are responsible for the life and death of their parents. They might think that, if mom or dad is not getting better, it's because they don't love mom or dad enough. The conclusion from this thought process is that they are a very bad person because they cannot love mom or dad enough to make them better.

All of these fears and anxieties can affect the child's behavior. Either the child may pretend that he doesn't care, or the child can be over-anxious to please.

The child who pretends not to care may be violent or aggressive. This might be interpreted as a way of saying "It's not my fault." It might also be a way of provoking the parent into anger and so making him or her more alive.

The child who is always very anxious to please is always very helpful and afraid of doing the wrong thing. He is almost doing a role reversal. Instead of being the child who needs to be cared for, he tries to be the parent.

These deep-down fears and anxieties need to be brought out into the open if the child is not going to be disturbed. Ideally, this needs to be done with a professional therapist or counselor.

WHO CARES FOR THE CARERS?

A new social problem has been highlighted recently in the UK by the Association of Carers—children caring for their disabled parents. If the able-bodied parent has to go out to work or has walked out on the family, it is not that unusual for some of the burden of care to fall on a child.

Even though in the UK there are social services, their first question is often to ask, "Isn't there somebody in the family who can help?" Rather than send round a home helper or a social worker to relieve the family, they leave it to the child or children in the family. Even children well under the age of majority are considered "somebody in the family" as far as helping a disabled person is concerned.

It is not unusual to find children as young as seven or eight doing the shopping, helping with the cooking, helping with the housework, and taking their disabled parent to the toilet in the night—all of this on top of going to school and doing homework.

In situations such as these, the child in question is often faced with a triple trauma: one parent has MS and is ill; the other parent has walked out because of this; and the child cannot do what normal children do because he or she has to do household and nursing duties. Children in situations such as this cannot go out to play with other children because they feel that they cannot leave the disabled parent alone—in case they need to go to the toilet, in case something happens, in case they need something.

This forces quite young children to be grown up before they have finished their childhood. It may make them into mature, helpful, altruistic adults, but it could also leave them resentful that they are sacrificing what they *really want* to do for something they really *don't want* to do.

As the years roll by, the child turns into a teenager and then a young adult. At this point, the disabled parent often feels a terrible burden on his own child—that he is getting in the way of that child leading a social life, going out and enjoying himself, even meeting someone and getting married.

None of these problems have easy solutions, and each individual situation will be different. Generally, the more help you can get from other people, the less likely it is that the children will have to bear an undue burden on their own.

THE PROBLEMS FOR PARENTS IF THEIR CHILD HAS MS

Of course, the situation can often be the other way around—the child (of whatever age) has MS, and the parent has to face that tragedy. How can you help your parents accept your illness without any feeling of guilt on their part or blame on your part?

If you think that there was something they did or did not do during your first fifteen or so years of life, you can easily feel that it's your parents' fault that you have MS. Maybe your mother fed you the wrong diet, maybe one of your parents passed on some genetic predisposition. Thoughts such as these may very well enter your mind. All of these thoughts are likely to be going through the parent's head as well: "If only I had done/not done this or that, this might never have happened."

The blame/guilt feelings may very well affect the relationship between the MS sufferer and his or her parents. Even if those actual emotions never come out into the open, they are still there, festering underneath.

If the person develops MS before he or she has found a partner and gotten married, it may fall on the parents to look after that child long after childhood is over. All parents want the best for their child and want to care for him as much as they can. The problems arise when the child is no longer a child but a young adult who wants independence from his parents and who does not want to be babied.

Being looked after by your parents once you are grown up is very demoralizing for some people. People do not want to be infantilized. For some people, this fear of being treated like a baby is worse than the fear of the disease itself.

Proving to your parents that you really *can* do things for yourself, that you really can manage on your own (if that's what you want to do) is one of the hardest things. Independence, perhaps in a specially adapted apartment, might be a better alternative than being treated like a child by your parents in the family home. However, it is particularly hard on the parents to have any peace of mind knowing that their son or daughter is alone in an apartment, possibly in real need of help.

Again, there are no easy solutions. Therapy or counseling may be vital to bring fears and deep emotions out into the open.

SEXUAL PROBLEMS IN MEN AND WOMEN

There is no reason why MS should stop or limit your sexual relationship with your partner or prevent you from being a person with sexual desires or needs. It is true that MS can cause specific sexual problems but, with love, information, communication, an open attitude, patience, and perhaps the help of new positions or sexual aids, these can be overcome.

If you are the one with MS, it is very important that your partner goes on seeing you as a sexually attractive person, and you must do everything to keep yourself that way. If you think you are unattractive or doubt your ability to attract or keep a partner, this will have a devastating effect on your self-image or self-esteem. It is vital to accept and love yourself so that others can feel that way about you too.

Your definition of sexuality may have to be broadened beyond the ability or inability just to have sexual intercourse.

To overcome sex problems, you have to communicate openly and honestly with your partner. If you do not share your feelings, your partner may not be aware of your needs. Love and patience on the part of both partners seldom fails to solve problems.

The worst thing you can do is avoid sexual contact. Some couples have a tendency to do this because they are afraid that sex will worsen the condition of the one with MS. On the other hand, they may avoid sex because they do not want it to end in disappointment or frustration, if this has been the outcome of previous encounters.

The danger is that, if you become too watchful or worried about what might go wrong, this "spectatoring" in itself becomes a problem. Performance anxieties always interfere with relaxation and enjoyment and can inhibit an erection in men and orgasm in women.

Fatigue

This is a major problem for both men and women with MS. However, it is possible to counteract fatigue being a sex problem if you plan your sex life beforehand, even though this does mean that sex will not be spontaneous.

Choose a time of day for sex when your energy is at its highest. It is silly to have sex late at night when you have no energy left. If you make love during the day, rest beforehand. If necessary, get your neighbors to take the children. Avoid interruptions. Try to create a relaxing and erotic atmosphere; this will help make the sexual encounter more satisfying.

Problems in Men

It is more likely to be men than women who complain of sexual dysfunction when they have MS. Any erection disturbance can make the sex act impossible; for women, sex is still possible despite any loss of feeling.

It has been estimated that 60 percent of men with MS do suffer from erection disturbances at some time in the disease, although emotional factors are thought to play a part in about 25 percent of these cases. About 25 percent of men with MS do become impotent. Remember that these statistics do not take into account the possibility of stabilizing the disease with the self-help methods described in this book. Like any other MS symptoms, potency can go away and then come back again. The range of symptoms in men can be anything from minor difficulties in getting and keeping an erection, to disturbances of sensation and ejaculation, to total failure to get an erection.

Ejaculation may be affected because it is a reflex controlled by the bundle of nerves in the lower spinal cord. Men who have difficulty getting or keeping an erect penis may be less likely to ejaculate.

It is possible for men to be given penile implants, which make the penis erect all the time and which make intercourse possible. There are also certain drugs that give erections which a man can inject into himself.

Men with MS who want to father children may be able to use a technique that involves the artificial stimulation of the penis to ejaculation. The wife is then a candidate for artificial insemination by husband (AIH). Unfortunately, this technique is not available in the UK, but it is in the USA.

Problems in Women

Women with MS may suffer loss of orgasm, diminished libido, or spasticity. They may also have problems with reduced lubrication, anxiety about bladder control, and fatigue. On the other hand, many women with quite severe disability do not experience any of these things and enjoy normal, satisfying sex.

Intercourse may be more difficult because of spasms of the thighs and reduced vaginal lubrication. An artificial lubricant, like KY Jelly, usually solves this.

Many women with MS continue to have a normal orgasm reflex. Others, depending on the extent of their neurological damage, may not experience genital orgasm. It is thought, however, that women who do not have a physiological orgasm can nevertheless reach a psychological climax—a sort of "phantom orgasm" following the partner's excitement and sharing a common tension release.

There is a definite connection between sexual problems and incontinence. Women tend to be anxious about bladder control when they are having sex. The same bundle of nerves that affects bladder control also controls the orgasm reflex. Women can be afraid of wetting themselves during intercourse or at orgasm. They may feel that they have to urinate while in the act of lovemaking. All of these things can stop you from letting yourself go.

Overcoming Sexual Problems

Even though sexual intercourse may be hard to achieve, many people find its emotional and psychological pleasure to be vital to a relationship. For this reason, it is worth striving to overcome specific difficulties.

If a man has erection difficulties, intercourse can be achieved by the woman sitting astride her partner and placing his flaccid penis inside her vagina. If she voluntarily contracts her vaginal muscles around his penis, she can hopefully bring about a partial erection.

It may be necessary to try new and different positions to accommodate the partner's specific problems. It should be possible to find a position that is comfortable and gives pleasure and satisfaction to both partners.

Catheters can be taped against the body so that they are out of the way. A man can wear a condom for hygiene.

If intercourse is too difficult, there are other sexual possibilities to maintain intimacy with your partner. Anything that gives mutual pleasure should be considered right and good, despite some people's attitudes that some practices might be "perverted." These would include oral sex, masturbation, and of course massaging, cuddling, fondling, or any other means of touching and mutual caressing. In a healthy sexual relationship, these would all be additions to sexual intercourse and not alternatives.

Sexual aids can give pleasure and satisfaction in lovemaking, so you should not treat them with suspicion just because they are manufactured and not "natural." Anything that does not actually cause pain in sex and that gives pleasure to both partners should be welcomed rather than shunned. After all, no one minds wearing glasses if their eyesight is poor; the same attitude should apply to sexual aids.

If you are embarrassed by the prospect of going into a sex shop, such items can be obtained by mail order.

Where to Go for Help with Sexual Problems

Counseling and plain information can make a big difference between a miserable sex life and a pleasurable one. There is a group in the United States that consults in daily living for the physically disabled:

SHARE (Sexuality Has A Right Everywhere)
Patricia Perlman
P.O. Box 188
Palisades Park, NJ 07650

Other Help

A husband, wife, or parent is probably not the best person to turn to. After all, they are suffering too, with similar feelings of loss, grief and fear. Cry together—but not on their shoulders. It does not always follow that the "unaffected" partner is the strong one. So it is better to turn to someone outside the immediate situation.

It is important that you do pour your heart out to somebody.

The worst thing that you can do is to bottle it up inside yourself—that would only add to your anxiety.

It is a good idea to have the safety valve of someone completely removed from your home situation. Someone you have never met before or a faceless voice on the telephone may be the best way for you to open up.

The National MS Society has peer counselors in some chapters, as already mentioned. Contact their Information Resource Center at 1-800-227-3166.

Psychotherapists

If you find yourself overwhelmed by depression as a result of having MS, your doctor should be able to refer you to a good psychotherapist. Even though psychotherapy is very time-consuming and can go on for years, it is worth considering if your personal relationship with your partner or any other problem is giving you distress and you are unable to sort it out all on your own.

Finally, it is worth saying again that many people with MS who have followed the various ways of managing the disease have not gotten worse and have lived virtually normal personal lives, becoming happy and fulfilled mothers and fathers able to lead normal family lives.

19

Childbirth and Children

Women with MS thinking of having a baby usually worry about having a relapse as a result. Instead of fearing the worst that having a baby might mean, you could perhaps dream about the best—the sheer joy that a baby brings.

"Joy" is a word that you hear over and over again when women talk about children. I know several women with MS who have had babies since their MS was diagnosed. In some, the MS has gotten worse since having their children. In others, it hasn't. Even those who are quite badly disabled do not regret for one moment that they had children. It would be a greater cause for regret if a woman decided against having children because she has MS.

CAN A WOMAN WITH MS HAVE CHILDREN?

One of the most pressing questions facing a young woman with MS is "Can I have children?" The answer, judging from the many thousands of women with MS who have happily had children, is a definite *yes*.

The "Baby M" Case

Some doctors in the USA are recommending that their female patients with MS not have a baby because there is a risk of a relapse as a result. In the famous "Baby M" case, a professional woman with only mild MS wanted to pay a surrogate mother to have a baby for her. She gave MS as the reason that she could not have a baby herself.

I cannot agree that MS is a good reason not to have a baby yourself. Speaking as a mother, I cannot imagine that a surrogate baby can feel the same to you as one you have carried and delivered yourself.

The "Baby M" case may have left the idea in the minds of many young women with MS that they cannot have a baby *because* they have MS. This is a tragic idea to give women who would dearly love to have a baby of their own. This book strongly takes the view that a woman with MS *can* have a baby.

Risks for Women with MS Who Become Pregnant

Some doctors say that having a baby when a woman has MS is not so much a medical problem as a social problem. By that, they mean that questions like "Who is going to look after the baby?" and "How much help and support can the husband give?" are more important than the physical side of childbirth, which doesn't in itself cause too many problems.

The risk time for women with MS is not during pregnancy or even during the delivery itself. It is after the baby is born— sometimes many months after, when the broken nights, constant demands of the infant, and tiredness can take their toll. That's why a mother with MS needs more support than normal, from husband, other members of the family, or paid help, so the risk of relapse is reduced.

Fertility

If you are healthy enough to have periods and healthy enough to get pregnant, then the chances are that you are healthy enough to have a baby successfully. Some women with MS lose their periods intermittently and are unable to get pregnant at those times. Overall, however, fertility is not thought to be affected.

If the man has MS, there may be problems in maintaining an

erection, in ejaculation, or both. Again, these problems can be intermittent. Many men with MS have fathered children since their MS was diagnosed. (See Chapter 18.)

Pregnancy

Once you have become pregnant, the pregnancy poses no special problems. Many women feel wonderfully well while they are pregnant, once the morning sickness phase has passed. Some of the symptoms during pregnancy may be perfectly normal and have nothing to do with MS, so don't get unduly worried if, for example, you want to dash to the bathroom more than usual.

The ARMS Research Unit at the Central Middlesex Hospital in London has been conducting some informal research about MS and childbirth. They followed thirteen pregnant women who passed through the unit. These women seemed to have fewer exacerbations of their MS during the second half of the pregnancy than would be expected.

The ARMS Unit also looked at the available research on the subject and came to the conclusion that pregnancy may actually *delay* relapses. This may possibly be due to a suppressive effect of alpha-fetoprotein, a substance found in the blood of pregnant women.

If someone did have an attack while they were pregnant, they might well think that their MS began or got worse because of the pregnancy. In fact, the figures seem to show that relapses and onset of MS during pregnancy occur no more often than would be expected in young women of childbearing age. It seems safe to say that relapses of MS are not caused by pregnancy.

Pre-Natal Care

There is no reason why you should not follow the same prenatal care as any other pregnant woman. Some obstetricians put women with MS into the "high risk" category and may therefore make you more anxious than need be. The things that make a woman "high risk" obstetrically have nothing to do with MS (e.g., high blood pressure, diabetes, obesity, etc.).

Your main problem during the pre-natal period will be resisting medically trained people who will try to persuade you to have a high tech birth, whether you want to or not. Decide what kind of birth you want early in the pregnancy, and make it clear to your hospital pre-natal clinic what you do and don't want.

During the pre-natal period, you might like to join a class of like-minded people for support and to make new friends who will then have babies the same age as yours.

If you do want a high tech birth, the best thing is to sign on at your hospital pre-natal clinic. If you have leanings toward natural childbirth, you could join La Leche League. For your local chapter of La Leche League, write to:

La Leche League International
9616 Minneapolis Avenue
Franklin Park, IL 60131

Can You Take Vitamins, Minerals, and Other Supplements during Pregnancy?
If you were taking evening primrose oil capsules plus vitamin and mineral supplements before you got pregnant, it is important not to change anything nutritionally either while you are pregnant or during breastfeeding. It would be unwise to start taking high doses of vitamins and minerals during the pregnancy unless you continue with these during breastfeeding, as the baby will get used to these high levels and could suffer from a sudden drop if you stopped taking them abruptly. Supplements of all of the B vitamins plus zinc at 15 mg twice a day would be useful to take during pregnancy.

Not only is it perfectly safe to take evening primrose oil during pregnancy, it may also be a way of protecting the baby from developing MS later in life. This may sound like an outrageous claim, but there may well be something in it. It is a hypothesis that can neither be proved nor disproved. (See the section on protecting your baby against getting MS, later in the chapter.)

Drugs during Pregnancy

This book takes the view that drugs that suppress the immune system are positively harmful. The whole book takes a nondrug approach to the management of MS, and this includes pregnancy and childbirth. Any drug can be dangerous during pregnancy, particularly in the first eleven weeks or so.

Drugs that you may have been taking before conception, such as prednisolone, ACTH, baclofen, Valium, or Dantrium, should be stopped before trying for a baby. The same applies to drugs used for urinary frequency or incontinence such as Cetiprin or Urispas. Long-term therapies such as azothioprine, cyclosporin, and even HBO should all be discontinued before conception.

The Delivery

When you go into labor, the contractions of the uterus are reflex actions, and MS does not affect them. The only problem is that childbirth can be tiring. What kind of delivery you have may depend on the severity of your MS. Unless you are very incapacitated, you have the same choices open to you as any other woman.

If you want a natural childbirth, with no drugs or interference, your biggest problem will probably be finding an obstetrician or a midwife who will agree to you having such a birth. Unless you are very lucky, most obstetricians and midwives are likely to classify you as "high risk" or "complicated." They are very likely to suggest that you have epidural anesthesia or even a planned cesarean section.

These obstetricians who like all their MS patients to have cesareans feel that the uterine muscles of a woman with MS may not be able to push the baby out without help. I do not know of any evidence that uterine muscles are affected by MS or any other kind of paraplegia. A cesarean is a fairly major operation, involving anesthetic and post-operative pain. As the mother, you are also denied the experience of actually giving birth yourself.

Most hospital births will involve a fair amount of technology. You are likely to be connected to a fetal heart monitor, with bands around your tummy connected to the monitoring machine. This means that you have to lie still during labor, instead of getting into any position you feel like. The fetal heart monitor is to detect whether the baby is getting into distress—but there are other ways of doing this.

The epidural will deaden the pain of the contractions, but it will also deaden feeling anything else from the waist downward. Someone with MS may find this particularly frightening because the loss of feeling might be MS and not just the anesthetic.

In a conventional hospital delivery, you would be given an intravenous drip. A hollow tube is inserted into a vein, which gives you a steady supply of dextrose to keep your strength up. Recent research has shown that this can actually *increase* your sensitivity to pain.

It is also quite likely that your delivery will be induced. At the time of the delivery, forceps may well be used, especially if the labor is induced and you have an epidural. Episiotomy—a cut to widen the vaginal opening—often goes with a forceps delivery.

Such a delivery—if you are not having a cesarean on the operating table—is almost certain to take place on a high delivery bed under bright lights. The medical personnel would all be wearing masks and gowns.

In short, the birth of your baby would be a medical event. The doctors may be offering you these technological aids because they think your birth will be made easier, safer, and less painful. However, there are many women who have been through this kind of birth experience who have felt out of control, as if the baby were being extracted from them.

Natural Birth
If you want your baby's birth to be a normal personal, physiological, and emotional experience, you will have to be very insistent to find an obstetrician who will be prepared to take you on for a natural birth. In a natural childbirth, you trust your body and go along with your instincts. During contractions, you can choose any position you like—on all fours, lying down, lunging forward, being on your side, sitting—anything that feels

comfortable. For the delivery itself, you might choose an upright position, such as squatting, hanging squat, or sitting, so that the baby drops down and the descent of the baby is helped by gravity.

When a woman is not interfered with and not disturbed during labor, she is able to secrete the right hormones. These hormones are vital for her feeling of well-being. Some of the chemicals she produces are endorphins. As well as making you feel "high," endorphins also act as painkillers, a bit like morphine.

You do not need strong leg muscles to have a natural birth. You can use a chair or special birthing stool to take your weight. Even if you do squat, it is only for the last couple of contractions anyway. Someone could help you by supporting you under your arms while you squat.

Of course, there are no drugs whatsoever in a natural birth. The rates of forceps use and episiotomy are lower than in high tech births.

Drugs routinely used in high tech births do affect the baby, so that they are born more dopey than in a natural birth. Babies born after a natural birth are immediately more alert. This is a good reason in itself to avoid drugs during labor and delivery.

AFTER THE BABY IS BORN

Immediately after the baby is delivered, it should be given to the mother and they should be together for at least the first hour after birth. Ideally, the father should be there too. This is the optimal time for "bonding" to take place, which is vital for the relationship between mother and child and for the healthy development of the baby. Ideally, there should be skin-to-skin contact, so the baby should not be wrapped at this stage. During the first hour, the baby develops the senses of sight, sound, touch, taste, and smell, and it instinctively finds the mother's nipple and begins to suck. The risk time for a mother with MS is often much later, when she can become exhausted by looking after a new baby. This later period is when you must have support, so you can get enough rest and sleep.

Relapses Around the Time of Birth

There have been several studies concerning the effects of child-birth on the long-term future of women with MS. All of them confirm that there is no difference in long-term disability of women with no baby, with one baby, or with two or more babies.

When there is a relapse during the period surrounding birth, it is more often three to four months after the birth. The ARMS figures are that, of thirteen pregnant women passing through the ARMS Research Unit, seven had a relapse three to six months after the birth. Of these, all were back to their previous state within a year. One had a relapse when her child was twelve months old. All of these relapses involved relatively minor symptoms.

The large studies looking at women with MS and childbirth suggest that 40 to 50 percent of women have relapses within three to six months after the birth. Of these, 80 percent recover fully and 20 percent have some residual damage. This suggests that, within a year of the birth, nearly all of the post-natal relapses have been overcome and the mother's condition has returned to the situation before the pregnancy, as far as the MS is concerned. Remember that these figures do not reflect the possibility of being able to fend off relapses by the self-help methods described in this book.

Breastfeeding

When a woman is breastfeeding, she secretes the hormone prolactin. A high secretion of prolactin over a long period might be a way to help the immune system recover its previous state. Therefore, prolonged breastfeeding may prevent a relapse at three to four months. It is very important that the baby gets the mother's colostrum when it is first born. Colostrum is the secretion that precedes actual breast milk and may play a very important part in building up immunity in the baby.

Prolonged breastfeeding is also the best possible way of protecting the baby. This is the time when myelination is occurring. The baby needs specific essential fatty acids for the structure of the myelin to be properly constituted. This period is also when the immune system is reaching maturity.

Breastfeeding is pleasurable and makes the bond between mother and baby even closer and more loving.

If you have any problems with breastfeeding, the best counselors are from

Le Leche League International
9616 Minneapolis Avenue
Franklin Park, IL 60131

Looking after a Baby

People talking about having a baby when the mother has MS tend to concentrate on the processes of pregnancy, labor, and the birth itself. The most physically demanding thing about having a baby, however, is the work involved in looking after it.

Caring for a baby is a twenty-four-hour-a-day job. However you feed your baby, for the first few months you will have very disturbed nights, with only a few hours' sleep at a time. Babies are extremely demanding, and it doesn't get much easier as they grow older.

It is very difficult to do anything else at all with a new baby in the house. All this is very exhausting, even for someone who does not have MS. The joys of a baby are worth it all, but you do need practical help.

Before the baby arrives, make whatever arrangements are necessary to get extra help. This may involve family, friends, neighbors, or paid help.

In addition to human help, try to equip your home with as many labor-saving devices as you can afford—such as a washing machine and dryer, dishwasher, microwave oven, etc. Easing the practical side of having a baby may go along way to preventing a relapse. Meeting other new mothers will help by providing you a network of friends and a life outside the home.

If you do have a relapse while your baby is still dependent on you, try to avoid going into the hospital, as it would be traumatic for the baby to be separated from you. To spare the baby emotional damage, it would be better to stay at home and be nursed there than to leave your baby and be admitted to the hospital without him.

It is important to try to do everything possible to avoid a relapse. All of the therapies in this book have had some success in stabilizing MS and reducing attacks.

WILL THE BABY BE ALL RIGHT?

MS is estimated to be between five and twenty times more common among near relatives of someone with MS. MS is not hereditary, but there is a familial link. The fact that MS does run more commonly in families is not special to MS—it happens in many conditions, such as heart disease, hypertension, or cancer.

There is a genetic element in MS. Again, this is the case with many diseases. However, even those born with the familial predisposition to MS will not necessarily develop the symptoms of MS later in their lives. There probably has to be a factor X, or many factors, to act on the susceptible person for MS to manifest itself. There is almost certainly an environmental factor or factors involved.

It is realistic to say that there is an increased risk of a child developing MS later on if the mother has MS. There is less of a chance if the father has MS. MS is not like hemophilia, however—it is not inevitably passed from mother to child. The majority of offspring of mothers or fathers with MS never get the disease.

Is There Any Way of Protecting Your Child against Developing MS?

This is a highly controversial area, and one that arouses very strong emotions. According to Professor E. J. Field, who is presently at Warwick University, MS *can* be prevented. This claim is of course totally unproven and could not be proved without terrible ethical and practical difficulties anyway.

Professor Field's hypothesis is roughly as follows. People with the familial predisposition to MS have anomalies in certain cell membranes because of abnormalities in the way they handle essential fatty acids. These anomalies can be detected by using Field's diagnostic test for MS, the electrophoretic mobility test.

Recent research has shown that by increasing the amount of polyunsaturates in the diet, these abnormalities can be corrected within a matter of months. This means that polyunsaturates should be considered a treatment for MS. This treatment could be in the form of a high EFA diet, such as the ARMS or Swank diet, or supplementation with polyunsaturates such as evening primrose oil.

Just as polyunsaturates can be a treatment, so can they also be a prevention, according to Professor Field. He feels that, if the mother takes supplements of evening primrose oil throughout her entire pregnancy and also throughout the entire period of breastfeeding—which should be as long as possible—the baby will have a high level of essential fatty acids in his cell membranes and therefore will not show any anomalies. He will therefore be protected against developing MS later. This preventive method seems more sensible than doing nothing and then having the child tested once it is past babyhood.

Professor Field also questions the way babies are fed. Perhaps current infant feeding practices, particularly early weaning off the breast on to formulas containing cow's milk, may prepare the soil for MS to develop later.

Testing for MS

Professor Field is able to do a blood test on those children who have a close relative with MS. By submitting this blood sample to various tests, including the electrophoretic mobility test, Professor Field is able to find out whether the child has the familiar predisposition.

In some cases he has found that a child gives what he calls "an MS reading." This means not that the child actually has MS, but that he is a candidate if the unknown factors come into play.

Again, Professor Field recommends evening primrose oil capsules. He claims that, if children who show a positive reading take evening primrose oil, their anomalous cells will become normal.

It has been impossible to prove whether children can be prevented from getting MS in this way. Many parents whose child has shown a predisposition in the blood test have taken the precaution of adding evening primrose oil to their child's daily diet on the principle that it is unlikely to do any harm and might do some good. For the majority of parents whose children have been given the all-clear, the test itself is a great relief.

Can Children Develop MS in Childhood?

The standard answer to this is no, but there is mounting evidence that the real answer is yes. Neurologists are taught that MS is a disease of young adulthood and that MS cannot be diagnosed under the age of around sixteen. If someone younger than that presents with classic MS symptoms, the doctor has to call it something else at least for the time being.

In his work, Professor Field has found cases of children under the age of fourteen who have not only shown anomalous results in his diagnostic test, but who have also shown typical MS symptoms. His advice to families is to give gamma-linolenate, in the form of evening primrose oil capsules, which is able to correct anomalous chemistry in a matter of months. Rather than wait for full-blown MS symptoms to show themselves, anyone who suspects that their child has MS could give him or her evening primrose oil without any harmful effects.

Do We Already Have a Prevention for MS?

Professor Field says, "To prevent the disease now seems a rational prospect capable of being put to the test with relatively little expenditure." For a long time, Professor Field has been suggesting that there should be centers all over England so children who have a near relative with MS can be tested using Field's diagnostic tests. In this way, those predisposed to MS could be discovered early and given preventive treatment. Professor Field believes that the preventive treatment for MS is gamma-linolenate in the form of evening primrose oil capsules. I feel it is a great pity that this idea, which might avoid so much human misery, has fallen on deaf ears.

MY OWN STORY

My son Pascal was born in April 1985. Throughout the pregnancy (as now), I was taking evening primrose oil capsules plus all the vitamins, minerals, and trace elements listed in Chapters 7 and 8.

I started attending the pre-natal clinic at the local hospital but opted out when I was classified as "high risk" because I was having a first baby at thirty-eight and had MS. I continued my pre-natal care with an independent midwife, who came to see me at my home. I worked at my job in TV until the eighth month of the pregnancy.

Pascal was born at home. My labor lasted three hours. I had no medical intervention during the labor or delivery. The baby's heartbeats were monitored from time to time with a portable Sonicaid. For the delivery, I was in the "hanging squat" position. I was standing up, put my arms around my partner's neck and clasped my hands, and then dropped down into a low squat. This is one of the favored positions of Dr. Michel Odent, who also happens to be my baby's father.

I had no tear, no episiotomy, no post-natal depression. Pascal began sucking at the breast within the first hour and has never been separated from me at night. We all sleep together in a big bed. Pascal breastfed until he was three and a half. Even though he is weaned, and has his own bed in his own room, he still joins us in the middle of the night to sleep snuggled next to his parents.

From the day when Pascal was born, I have been lucky enough to have help in the house and with the baby. In the mornings, Laraine helps me with household chores and shopping as well as the baby. In the afternoons, Muriel plays with Pascal while I work. Without these two wonderful women, I doubt that I would be as well as I am today. Looking after a new baby, running a household, and working all at the same time can be very exhausting. I don't think I could have survived the exhaustion of it all without their help.

When Pascal was a few months old, I called Professor Field and asked him whether I should bring Pascal to be tested. When he heard that I had been taking evening primrose oil all through my pregnancy and also while breastfeeding, he said there would be no need—Pascal would be protected already, so the tests would be a waste of time.

Now Pascal eats the same food we do, which I haven't the heart to deny him. I am hoping that the long period of breastfeeding will have given him the best start in life, and that he will continue to be healthy.

For myself, my ambition is to continue being a healthy mother to Pascal.

Further Reading

Allergies—Your Hidden Enemy, Theron G. Randolph and Ralph W. Moss (Thorsons, 1984).

The ARMS EFA Diet (available from ARMS—see useful addresses, following).

By Appointment Only—Multiple Sclerosis, Jan De Vries (Mainstream Publishing).

Candida Albicans: Could Yeast Be Your Problem? Leon Chaitow (Healing Arts Press, 1985).

Clinical Ecology, George Lewith and Julian Kenyon (Thorsons, 1985).

Evening Primrose Oil, Judy Graham (Healing Arts Press, 1984).

Love, Medicine and Miracles, Bernie S. Siegel, M.D. (Harper & Row, 1986).

The Migraine Revolution, Dr. John Mansfield (Thorsons, 1986)—good for information on food allergies and chronic illness.

MS—Something Can Be Done and You Can Do It, Soll and Grenoble (Contemporary Books, 1984).

The Multiple Sclerosis Diet Book, Roy Swank, M.D., and Barbara Brewer Dugan (Doubleday, 1987).

Multiple Sclerosis in Childhood—Diagnosis and Prophylaxis, Professor E. J. Field (Charles C. Thomas, 1980).

The Natural Family Doctor, Dr. Andrew Stanway, general editor (Century, 1987).

Nutritional Medicine, Dr. Stephen Davies and Dr. Alan Stewart (Pan Books, 1987).

The Toxic Time Bomb, Sam Ziff (Thorsons, 1985).

21st Century Medicine, Dr. Julian Kenyon (Thorsons, 1986).

Vaccination and Immunisation: Dangers, Delusions and Alternatives, Leon Chaitow (C. W. Daniel, 1987).

The Yeast Connection, William G. Crook (Vintage Books, 1986).

Yoga for the Disabled, Howard Kent (Thorsons, 1985).

You Can Heal Your Life, Louise L. Hay (Hay House, 1984).

The Z Factor, Judy Graham and Michel Odent (Thorsons, 1986).

Newsletters

ARMS Link

Quarterly newsletter available free to ARMS members. Letters to the editor contain useful hints on how people manage their MS.

Multiple Sclerosis Newsletter
From the office of Professor Roy Swank:

Department of Neurology
Oregon Health Sciences University
3181 S.W. Sam Jackson Park Road
Portland, OR 97201

Very useful for advice on management of MS, hints on daily living, etc.

Inside MS
Published quarterly by the National Multiple Sclerosis Society

205 East 42nd Street
New York, NY 10017
Tel: 212-986-3240
or toll-free 1-800-624-8236

The People's Doctor Newsletter

PO Box 982
Evanston, IL 60204

Radical medical advice, not just on MS.

Useful Names and Addresses

HMS, Inc.
(Helping Multiple Sclerosis, Inc.)
Mr. Rudy Burger, Chairman & Founder
P.O. Box 1
Darien, CT 06820

The Jimmie Heuga Centre for People with Physical Challenges
P.O. Box 2289
Avon, CO 81620
Tel: 303-949-4922

Kaslow Medical Self-Care Centers
795 Alamo Pintado Road
Solvang, CA 93463
Tel: 805-688-5519
(A center that focuses on the connection between diet and disease.)

The Medical Rehabilitation Research and Training Center for Multiple
    Sclerosis
Albert Einstein College of Medicine
1300 Morris Park Avenue
Bronx, NY 10461
Tel: 212-430-2682

MS Roundhouse
7720 Sebago Road
Bethesda, MD 20817
Tel: 301-229-3027
(A psychological and educational treatment center for MS.)

Multiple Sclerosis Self Help Project
PO Box 7573
Berkeley, CA 94707
(publishes helpful newsletter)

National Multiple Sclerosis Society
205 East 42nd Street
New York, NY 10017
Tel: 212-986-3240
or toll free: 1-800-624-8236

Paula Rayman
The Mary Ingraham Bunting Institute
Radcliffe College
Ten Garden Street
Cambridge, MA 02138
Tel: 617-495-8212
(coordinates a self-help group of women with MS in Massachusetts)

Rocky Mountain Multiple Sclerosis Center
Dr. Jack Burks, Executive Director
University of Colorado Health Sciences Center
PO Box B181
4200 E. 9th Avenue
Denver, CO 80262
Tel: 303-394-8967
(A comprehensive center for the diagnosis, treatment, and rehabilita-
tion of individuals with MS.)

Professor Roy Swank (newsletter)
Department of Neurology
Oregon Health Sciences University
3181 S.W. Sam Jackson Park Road
Portland, OR 97201

Supplements

Evening primrose oil capsules are now manufactured by several
companies. The brand that has been the subject of most research
is Efamol, distributed in the United States by:

Nature's Way Products
P.O. Box 2233
Springville, UT 84663
Tel: 801-489-3635

Index

BOOKS OF RELATED INTEREST

MULTIPLE SCLEROSIS AND HAVING A BABY
Everything You Need to Know about Conception,
Pregnancy, and Parenthood
by Judy Graham

HEALING WITHOUT FEAR
How to Overcome Your Fear of Doctors, Hospitals, and the
Health Care System and Find Your Way to True Healing
by Laurel Ann Reinhardt, Ph.D.

VIBRATIONAL MEDICINE
The #1 Handbook of Subtle-Energy Therapies
by Richard Gerber, M.D.

THE COX-2 CONNECTION
Natural Breakthrough Treatment for Arthritis,
Alzheimer's, and Cancer
by James B. LaValle, R.Ph., N.M.D., C.C.N

GENETICALLY ENGINEERED FOOD:
CHANGING THE NATURE OF NATURE
What You Need to Know to Protect Yourself,
Your Family, and Our Planet
by Martin Teitel, Ph.D., and Kimberly A. Wilson

FOOD ALLERGIES AND FOOD INTOLERANCE
The Complete Guide to Their Identification and Treatment
by Jonathan Brostoff, M.D., and Linda Gamlin

LUPUS
Alternative Therapies That Work
by Sharon Moore

THE SEASONAL DETOX DIET
Remedies from the Ancient Cookfire
by Carrie L'Esperance

Inner Traditions • Bear & Company
P.O. Box 388 • Rochester, VT 05767
1-800-246-8648
www.InnerTraditions.com

Or contact your local bookseller